Asthma and Allergic Inflammation: Risks, Mechanisms, and New Treatments

Asthma and Allergic Inflammation: Risks, Mechanisms, and New Treatments

Editors

Luis Garcia-Marcos
Kostas N. Priftis

MDPI • Basel • Beijing • Wuhan • Barcelona • Belgrade • Manchester • Tokyo • Cluj • Tianjin

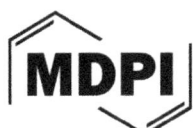

Editors
Luis Garcia-Marcos
University of Murcia
Spain

Kostas N. Priftis
National and Kapodistrian University of Athens
Greece

Editorial Office
MDPI
St. Alban-Anlage 66
4052 Basel, Switzerland

This is a reprint of articles from the Special Issue published online in the open access journal *Journal of Clinical Medicine* (ISSN 2077-0383) (available at: https://www.mdpi.com/journal/jcm/special_issues/Asthma_Allergic_Inflammation).

For citation purposes, cite each article independently as indicated on the article page online and as indicated below:

LastName, A.A.; LastName, B.B.; LastName, C.C. Article Title. *Journal Name* **Year**, *Volume Number*, Page Range.

ISBN 978-3-0365-2141-1 (Hbk)
ISBN 978-3-0365-2142-8 (PDF)

Cover image courtesy of Luis Garcia-Marcos

© 2021 by the authors. Articles in this book are Open Access and distributed under the Creative Commons Attribution (CC BY) license, which allows users to download, copy and build upon published articles, as long as the author and publisher are properly credited, which ensures maximum dissemination and a wider impact of our publications.

The book as a whole is distributed by MDPI under the terms and conditions of the Creative Commons license CC BY-NC-ND.

Contents

About the Editors vii

Luis García-Marcos
What Is Asthma?
Reprinted from: *J. Clin. Med.* **2021**, *10*, 1282, doi:10.3390/jcm10061282 1

John O. Warner
Asthma/Rhinitis (The United Airway) and Allergy: Chicken or Egg; Which Comes First?
Reprinted from: *J. Clin. Med.* **2020**, *9*, 1483, doi:10.3390/jcm9051483 5

Philippa Ellwood, Eamon Ellwood, Charlotte Rutter, Virginia Perez-Fernandez, Eva Morales, Luis García-Marcos, Neil Pearce, M Innes Asher, David Strachan and on behalf of the GAN Phase I Study Group
Global Asthma Network Phase I Surveillance: Geographical Coverage and Response Rates
Reprinted from: *J. Clin. Med.* **2020**, *9*, 3688, doi:10.3390/jcm9113688 17

Sara Maio, Sandra Baldacci, Marzia Simoni, Anna Angino, Stefania La Grutta, Vito Muggeo, Salvatore Fasola, Giovanni Viegi and on behalf of the AGAVE Pisa Group
Longitudinal Asthma Patterns in Italian Adult General Population Samples: Host and Environmental Risk Factors
Reprinted from: *J. Clin. Med.* **2020**, *9*, 3632, doi:10.3390/jcm9113632 35

Carmen Frontela-Saseta, Carlos A. González-Bermúdez and Luis García-Marcos
Diet: A Specific Part of the Western Lifestyle Pack in the Asthma Epidemic
Reprinted from: *J. Clin. Med.* **2020**, *9*, 2063, doi:10.3390/jcm9072063 51

Manuel Sanchez-Solis, Maria Soledad Parra-Carrillo, Pedro Mondejar-Lopez, Patricia W Garcia-Marcos and Luis Garcia-Marcos
Preschool Asthma Symptoms in Children Born Preterm: The Relevance of Lung Function in Infancy
Reprinted from: *J. Clin. Med.* **2020**, *9*, 3345, doi:10.3390/jcm9103345 67

Giulia Scioscia, Giovanna Elisiana Carpagnano, Donato Lacedonia, Piera Soccio, Carla Maria Irene Quarato, Luigia Trabace, Paolo Fuso and Maria Pia Foschino Barbaro
The Role of Airways 17β-Estradiol as a Biomarker of Severity in Postmenopausal Asthma: A Pilot Study
Reprinted from: *J. Clin. Med.* **2020**, *9*, 2037, doi:10.3390/jcm9072037 75

Alan Kaplan, Patrick D. Mitchell, Andrew J. Cave, Remi Gagnon, Vanessa Foran and Anne K. Ellis
Effective Asthma Management: Is It Time to Let the AIR out of SABA?
Reprinted from: *J. Clin. Med.* **2020**, *9*, 921, doi:10.3390/jcm9040921 85

Carlo Caffarelli, Carla Mastrorilli, Michela Procaccianti and Angelica Santoro
Use of Sublingual Immunotherapy for Aeroallergens in Children with Asthma
Reprinted from: *J. Clin. Med.* **2020**, *9*, 3381, doi:10.3390/jcm9103381 95

Andrew Bush
Which Child with Asthma is a Candidate for Biological Therapies?
Reprinted from: *J. Clin. Med.* **2020**, *9*, 1237, doi:10.3390/jcm9041237 111

Konstantinos Douros, Olympia Sardeli, Spyridon Prountzos, Angeliki Galani, Dafni Moriki, Efthymia Alexopoulou and Kostas N. Priftis
Asthma-Like Features and Anti-Asthmatic Drug Prescription in Children with Non-CF Bronchiectasis
Reprinted from: *J. Clin. Med.* **2020**, *9*, 4009, doi:10.3390/jcm9124009 . . . . **127**

About the Editors

Luis Garcia-Marcos is Professor of Paediatrics, Chair at the University of Murcia and leads the research of the Pulmonology and Allergy Units at the "Arrixaca" Children's University Hospital in Murcia, Spain. He also served as vice-director of the Bio-Health Research Institute of Murcia (IMIB-Arrixaca) and as vice president of Health Sciences at the University of Murcia. He obtained his degree in Medicine at the University of Valencia, Spain, and was trained as a paediatrician in his current hospital and in the London Hospital for Sick Children at Great Ormond Street, UK. His PhD was issued by the University of Murcia. He has been a research scholar at the Arizona Respiratory Center and the BIO5 Institute, University of Arizona, Tucson, (AZ, USA). He is also an Associated Professor of Paediatrics at the University of Santiago, Chile. His main research interests are the epidemiology of allergic diseases, including asthma, and the lung function of infants. He served as a member of the steering and executive committees of the International Study of Asthma and Allergies in Childhood (ISAAC) collaboration for the last 7 years, and is a member of the steering committee for the Global Asthma Network (GAN). He has been the editor of "Allergologia et Immunopathologia" since 2008, and has served in different task forces and committees of the European Respiratory Society.

Kostas N. Priftis is a Professor of Paediatric Respiratory Medicine at the National and Kapodistrian Athens University (NKUA) Medical School in Athens, Greece. He graduated from medical school at the Aristotle University of Thessaloniki, defended his PhD thesis at the NKUA Medical School, completed paediatric training at the University of Patras and obtained a research fellowship in paediatric respiratory medicine at the Children's Respiratory Unit of the University of Nottingham Medical School, UK.

His research is focused on childhood asthma, paediatric bronchoscopy, chronic endobronchial infections, breath sounds and allergy. He has more than 180 scientific publications in peer-reviewed international journals and has edited eight books and special issues. He founded the two-year Master's program in Paediatric Respiratory Medicine at NKUA Medical School.

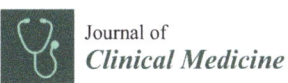

Editorial

What Is Asthma?

Luis García-Marcos [1,2,3]

1. Paediatric Allergy and Pulmonology Units, 'Virgen de la Arrixaca' University Children's Hospital, University of Murcia, 30100 Murcia, Spain; lgmarcos@um.es
2. Biomedical Research Institute of Murcia (IMIB-Arrixaca), 30120 Murcia, Spain
3. Network of Asthma and Adverse and Allergic Reactions (ARADyAL), 28029 Madrid, Spain

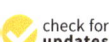

Citation: García-Marcos, L. What Is Asthma?. *J. Clin. Med.* **2021**, *10*, 1282. https://doi.org/10.3390/jcm1006 1282

Received: 12 March 2021
Accepted: 16 March 2021
Published: 19 March 2021

Publisher's Note: MDPI stays neutral with regard to jurisdictional claims in published maps and institutional affiliations.

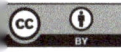

Copyright: © 2021 by the author. Licensee MDPI, Basel, Switzerland. This article is an open access article distributed under the terms and conditions of the Creative Commons Attribution (CC BY) license (https://creativecommons.org/licenses/by/4.0/).

Asthma is . . . . what? A symptom, a condition, a disease? I have been speaking about asthma and I have been hearing about asthma for the last 40 years. I have heard about allergy and about phenotypes in children and in adults; I have also heard of endotypes and even of "other-types". I come from the time that having a space mask was a privilege and now I have to decide what biological therapy is better for a specific child and to "tailor" a treatment following the guidelines of the Lancet commission [1]. Things seem to have changed very much, but, in essence, asthma remains a mystery. Maybe because, as Fernando Martínez reminded us some time ago, asthma is now like fever was in the late 19th century, which was considered a disease [2].

Thus, it is also a good idea to dedicate some discussion to asthma and the new achievements related to the disease, but also to the old paradigms of this condition . . . or should I have said symptom? The *Journal of Clinical Medicine* had the good idea of launching a Special Issue on asthma, but the not so good one of asking me to organize it. Anyhow, good friends ("that's what friends are for", as Dionne Warwick put it) decided to accompany me in this task and contribute with their knowledge.

John Warner decided to revisit an old but never solved question about the commencement of humanity—the egg or the chicken [3]—and, in masterful fashion, he led us from the basics to personalized treatment, taking into account the so-called "allergic march". Andy Bush, always on the cutting edge of knowledge, explains to us what child is a good candidate for biological therapy and revisits the need to establish phenotypes (which maybe not be as stable as we would like them) to make better decisions [4]. Phenotypes (in adults) are also the topic of the paper by Sara Maio and the AGAVE Pisa group [5]. They very elegantly show, through latent transition analysis, that some environmental factors are crucial for defining some phenotypes and even that there may be specific forms of asthma associated to tobacco smoke or air pollution.

Alan Kaplan and colleagues [6] suggest, with all of my support, that it is time to shift to SABA-ICS reliever medication, and I would also add in Paediatrics. In this same department of general treatment, Carlo Caffarelli and colleagues [7] update the usage of sublingual immunotherapy in children. This somewhat different approach to immunotherapy for asthma has still some detractors, but seems to be becoming adept as evidence accumulates that it is a good option when the right patient is chosen . . . or perhaps I should put it the other way around: when the patient meets the criteria for its indication.

My good friend and colleague Manuel Sánchez-Solis continues the saga of lung development in the early stages and later asthma with new data on children born prematurely [8] and elegantly shows that a limited lung function during infancy is a risk of future wheezing and of severe wheezing episodes. I think we forget about lung maturation when dealing with asthma and it is quite probable that, in a totally separate path of the TH2 one, ill-matured lungs are much more prone to asthma symptoms in childhood and even later on than correctly matured lungs. Lung development and maturing is probably the reason why preterm birth is a risk for asthma and, as showed by Vogt et al., every week (of gestation) counts [9].

In addition, what about the markers? We desperately need markers of asthma and of asthma phenotypes. Especially, early markers of the condition which might point to primary prevention measures. After the tailored treatments this is, in my opinion, the way we should go if we want to really diminish the burden of asthma. In this Special Issue, Giulia Scioscia and her Italian colleagues [10] add another brick to the wall and show that estradiol in airways may well be a good marker of postmenopausal severe asthma and help to phenotype severe asthmatic patients with neutrophil inflammation.

In the epidemiology arena, Carmen Frontela and colleagues [11] indirectly put the focus on another forgotten road to asthma that has not been sufficiently insisted on: oxidative stress. Yes, it is not a pathway as explored and consistent as the Th2 one, but there is already enough evidence that mechanisms related to the handling of free radicals have a role in asthma [12]. However, there is also obesity and its double adverse effects on lungs: the low-level inflammation and the usually forgotten relationship with the lack of enough exercise and the need to stretch bronchial muscles to have then well developed and "in good shape" in order to avoid over-contraction [13]. Did I mention that this is part of the Western lifestyle package?

This Special Issue has also the privilege and the honor of including the first results from the Global Asthma Network (GAN) Phase I study [14]. Its predecessor, the International Study of Asthma and Allergies in Childhood (ISAAC), made possible in great part by some of the authors of this paper, namely, Innes Asher, Philippa Ellwood, Neil Pearce and David Strachan, was an enormous breakthrough in asthma epidemiology in children. GAN also includes the adult population. I am sure this paper is the starting gun of a new story which promises to be fascinating.

This Special Issue is probably not going to solve the problem, but will be interesting to read as it contains valuable information of almost every part of the asthma spectrum. It is the job of the reader to try and put the pieces in the right place (if there is a right place) to try and get a world envisioned by the Global Asthma Network where "no-one suffers from asthma".

Oops ... also, as warned by the Greek friends [15], please do not confound asthma with bronchiectasis ... or have some patients with bronchiectasis symptoms of asthma?... So, then ... what is asthma?

Funding: This research received no external funding.

Conflicts of Interest: The authors declare no conflict of interest.

References

1. Pavord, I.D.; Beasley, R.; Agusti, A.; Anderson, G.P.; Bel, E.; Brusselle, G.; Cullinan, P.; Custovic, A.; Ducharme, F.M.; Fahy, J.V.; et al. After asthma: Redefining airways diseases. *Lancet* **2018**, *391*, 350–400. [CrossRef]
2. Harding, A. Fernando Martinez: Seeking to solve the puzzle of asthma. *Lancet* **2006**, *368*, 725. [CrossRef]
3. Warner, J.O. Asthma/Rhinitis (The United Airway) and Allergy: Chicken or Egg; Which Comes First? *J. Clin. Med.* **2020**, *9*, 1483. [CrossRef] [PubMed]
4. Bush, A. Which Child with Asthma is a Candidate for Biological Therapies? *J. Clin. Med.* **2020**, *9*, 1237. [CrossRef] [PubMed]
5. Maio, S.; Baldacci, S.; Simoni, M.; Angino, A.; La Grutta, S.; Muggeo, V.; Fasola, S.; Viegi, G. Longitudinal Asthma Patterns in Italian Adult General Population Samples: Host and Environmental Risk Factors. *J. Clin. Med.* **2020**, *9*, 3632. [CrossRef] [PubMed]
6. Kaplan, A.; Mitchell, P.D.; Cave, A.J.; Gagnon, R.; Foran, V.; Ellis, A.K. Effective Asthma Management: Is It Time to Let the AIR out of SABA? *J. Clin. Med.* **2020**, *9*, 921. [CrossRef] [PubMed]
7. Caffarelli, C.; Mastrorilli, C.; Procaccianti, M.; Santoro, A. Use of Sublingual Immunotherapy for Aeroallergens in Children with Asthma. *J. Clin. Med.* **2020**, *9*, 3381. [CrossRef] [PubMed]
8. Sanchez-Solis, M.; Parra-Carrillo, M.S.; Mondejar-Lopez, P.; Garcia-Marcos, P.W.; Garcia-Marcos, L. Preschool Asthma Symptoms in Children Born Preterm: The Relevance of Lung Function in Infancy. *J. Clin. Med.* **2020**, *9*, 3345. [CrossRef] [PubMed]
9. Vogt, H.; Lindstrom, K.; Bråbäck, L.; Hjern, A. Preterm Birth and Inhaled Corticosteroid Use in 6- to 19-Year-Olds: A Swedish National Cohort Study. *Pediatrics* **2011**, *127*, 1052–1059. [CrossRef] [PubMed]
10. Scioscia, G.; Carpagnano, G.E.; Lacedonia, D.; Soccio, P.; Quarato, C.M.I.; Trabace, L.; Fuso, P.; Foschino Barbaro, M.P. The Role of Airways 17β-Estradiol as a Biomarker of Severity in Postmenopausal Asthma: A Pilot Study. *J. Clin. Med.* **2020**, *9*, 2037. [CrossRef] [PubMed]

11. Frontela-Saseta, C.; González-Bermúdez, C.A.; García-Marcos, L. Diet: A Specific Part of the Western Lifestyle Pack in the Asthma Epidemic. *J. Clin. Med.* **2020**, *9*, 2063. [CrossRef] [PubMed]
12. Sahiner, U.M.; Birben, E.; Erzurum, S.; Sackesen, C.; Kalayci, Ö. Oxidative stress in asthma: Part of the puzzle. *Pediatr. Allergy Immunol.* **2018**, *29*, 789–800. [CrossRef] [PubMed]
13. Alexander, C.J. Asthma: A disuse contracture? *Med. Hypotheses* **2005**, *64*, 1102–1104. [CrossRef] [PubMed]
14. Ellwood, P.; Ellwood, E.; Rutter, C.; Perez-Fernandez, V.; Morales, E.; Garcia-Marcos, L.; Pearce, N.; Asher, M.I.; Strachan, D. Global Asthma Network Phase I Surveillance: Geographical Coverage and Response Rates. *J. Clin. Med.* **2020**, *9*, 3688. [CrossRef] [PubMed]
15. Global Asthma Network. Available online: http://www.globalasthmanetwork.org/about/vision.php (accessed on 25 February 2021).

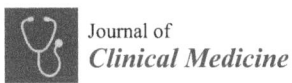

Review

Asthma/Rhinitis (The United Airway) and Allergy: Chicken or Egg; Which Comes First?

John O. Warner [1,2]

1. Emeritus Professor of Paediatrics, National Heart and Lung Institute, Imperial College, London SW3 6LY, UK; j.o.warner@imperial.ac.uk
2. Honorary Professor of Paediatrics, University of Cape Town, Cape Town 7701, Western Cape, South Africa

Received: 21 April 2020; Accepted: 11 May 2020; Published: 14 May 2020

Abstract: While allergy, asthma and rhinitis do not inevitably co-exist, there are strong associations. Not all those with asthma are allergic, rhinitis may exist without asthma, and allergy commonly exists in the absence of asthma and/or rhinitis. This is likely due to the separate gene/environment interactions which influence susceptibility to allergic sensitization and allergic airway diseases. Allergic sensitization, particularly to foods, and eczema commonly manifest early in infancy, and not infrequently are followed by the development of allergic rhinitis and ultimately asthma. This has become known as the "allergic march". However, many infants with eczema never develop asthma or rhinitis, and both the latter conditions can evolve without prior eczema or food allergy. Understanding the mechanisms underlying the ontogeny of allergic sensitization and allergic disease will facilitate rational approaches to the prevention and management of asthma and allergic rhinitis. Furthermore, a range of new, so-called biological, therapeutic approaches, targeting specific allergy-promoting and pro-inflammatory molecules, are now in clinical trials or have been recently approved for use by regulatory authorities and could have a major impact on disease prevention and control in the future. Understanding basic mechanisms will be essential to the employment of such medications. This review will explain the concept of the united airway (rhinitis/asthma) and associations with allergy. It will incorporate understanding of the role of genes and environment in relation to the distinct but interacting origins of allergy and rhinitis/asthma. Understanding the patho-physiological differences and varying therapeutic requirements in patients with asthma, with or without rhinitis, and with or without associated allergy, will aid the planning of a personalized evidence-based management strategy.

Keywords: asthma; rhinitis; allergy; allergic sensitization; genomics; epigenetics; hygiene hypothesis; allergic march; gene/environment interactions; personalized medicine

1. Introduction

There is a compelling list of evidence to support the concept that allergy is fundamental to persistent asthma. Allergy in the child and family is a risk factor for later rhinitis and asthma. Early onset allergy is a poor prognostic factor for those who subsequently develop asthma. Direct allergen exposure into the nose in allergically sensitized subjects will incite allergic rhinitis and inhaled into lower airways an asthmatic reaction. The severity of asthma is directly associated with the degree of allergy and with food allergy. Monoclonal anti-Immunoglobulin E (IgE) improves allergic asthma and allergen immunotherapy is the only treatment which modifies long-term outcomes for rhinitis and asthma. However, the attributable percentage of asthma due to allergy never reaches even 50%, and in some environments is less than 10%. The overall attributable fraction throughout Europe from one study, was 30%, but ranged between 4% and 61% between countries [1]. However, attribution varies with age, with allergy being more strongly related to asthma in children compared to adults.

The histopathology of asthma, and to a lesser extent allergic rhinitis, is characterized by airway inflammation, involving to a variable extent, neutrophils, eosinophils and mast-cells. However, the component most associated with persistent and more severe disease is airway remodeling, with increased collagen in the lamina reticularis (seen as apparent thickening of the basement membrane) and submucosa. There is also hypertrophy of smooth muscle and associated bronchial hyper-responsiveness (BHR). Many of these features sometimes manifest independent of allergy [2].

It is therefore necessary to re-evaluate the allergy/rhinitis/asthma relationships.

2. Gene/Environment Interactions

The genetics of rhinitis and asthma do not exhibit simple Mendelian inheritance. Many genes are involved, each having very small phenotypic effects. Gene polymorphisms have variously been associated with allergy, and/or asthma, and/or eczema, and/or rhinitis. It has therefore been suggested that it is more fruitful to focus on gene/environment interactions, epigenetics, and pharmaco-genetics [3].

Airway inflammation and bronchospasm can occur because of gene and environmental interactions, resulting in alterations in airway structure and function (airway dysmorphisms), independent of allergy (Figure 1). Changes in structure can modify the behavior of inflammatory cells and susceptibility to infection. Thus, polymorphisms in the A Disintegrin and Metalloprotease 33-ADAM 33 (20p13) and OrmDL3 (17q21) genes increase susceptibility to wheezing in infancy and possibly later-life Chronic Obstructive Pulmonary Disease—COPD, but not necessarily asthma. These genes are not expressed in immunologically active cells but are associated with influences on airway structure and function [4,5]. There is evidence that ADAM 33 polymorphisms result in airway remodeling in the presence of environmental triggers, and that this may even commence during fetal life [6]. A meta-analysis of genome-wide association studies has shown linkage with several genes on chromosome 17q21, including those coding for Thymic Stromal Lymphopoetin (TSLP) and Interleukin-33 (IL33), which are expressed in epithelial cells. When these cells are damaged, TSLP, IL25 and IL33 are released and stimulate release of IL4 from innate lymphocytic cells. This in turn facilitates the development of an adaptive T-helper lymphocyte type 2 (Th2) allergy promoting hypersensitivity [7]. Implicit from all the association studies is that asthma is heterogeneous with a range of genetic influences on airway morphology, and on signals from damaged epithelial cells which switch on an adaptive immune response leading to airway inflammation. These changes are not influenced by prior allergic sensitization but may contribute to its subsequent development [8].

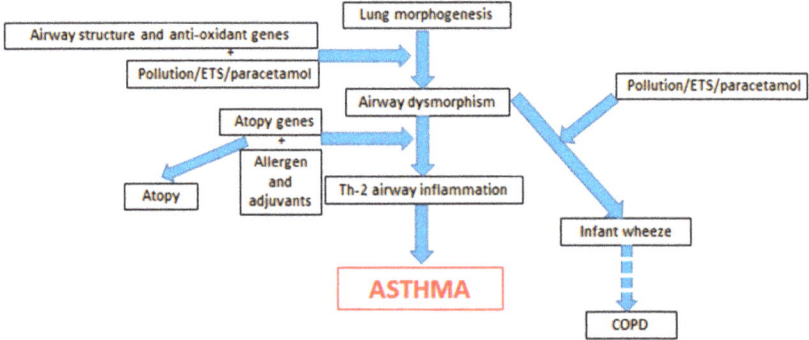

Figure 1. A schematic representation of the impact of timing of environmental interactions with genetic polymorphisms on the ontogeny of allergic sensitization and three wheeze phenotypes; infant wheeze, asthma and Chronic Obstructive Pulmonary Disease (COPD). ETS is environmental tobacco smoke.

Gene polymorphisms, which impair anti-oxidant activity, predispose to wheeze in the presence of early life environmental tobacco smoke (ETS) and other pollutant exposures, as well as airway infections, but are not necessarily associated with allergy [9]. Epidemiological studies have suggested that both maternal pregnancy and infant paracetamol exposure increase the risk of asthma [10,11]. A paracetamol metabolite, n-acetylbenzoquinonimine, depletes anti-oxidant activity, and one intriguing study suggests that there is an interaction, increasing the risk of wheeze at 5 years of age, between the number of days that pregnant women take this analgesic and a polymorphism in the Glutathione S-Transferase P-1 anti-oxidant gene [12]. Impairment of anti-oxidant activity will increase the risks of persistent airway inflammation in response to infection or pollutant exposure.

Separate gene polymorphisms affecting immune modulation predispose to allergic sensitization in the presence of allergen and adjuvant exposure. There are fewer genome-wide association studies of allergic sensitization alone compared with those for allergic diseases such as asthma and eczema. They have revealed a range of gene polymorphisms, associated with regulation of T-lymphocyte responses, IgE (the allergy antibody) production, and the IgE receptor [13]. Some are common to those associated with asthma, such as genes for TSLP and IL33, while others are independent, such as those in the cytokine gene cluster on 5q31-33 [14].

Variations in the genome (nature) have only small effects on allergy and airway phenotypes, and environment (nurture) clearly plays a greater part. Epigenetic phenomena explain much of the science underlying gene/environment interactions. These are changes to DNA expression without modification of DNA sequences. They occur by: methylation of DNA Cytosine-phosphodiesterase-Guanine CpG motifs (30 million in the human genome), which impairs transcription; histone modification, around which DNA is coiled, on 30 million nucleosomes by acetylation, methylation, phosphorylation, and ubiquitination, which opens chromatin to aid transcription; and microRNAs in the cytoplasm, which mostly block mRNA transcription. Many environmental factors have their influence through epigenetic effects. This has been best studied for CpG methylation [15]. Most notable is the effect of ETS and pollutant exposure, which have been shown to affect CpG methylation and histone modification [16]. While influences may occur at any age, epigenetic effects can be hereditable, and this has been demonstrated in a study of grand–mother ETS exposure which independently increased the risk of asthma in grand-children, irrespective of maternal smoking [17]. Even minor variations in diet can have epigenetic effects. Thus, folic acid—a methyl donor—supplementation during pregnancy has been associated with an increased risk of asthma in childhood [18].

Pharmaco-genetic studies have identified genetic variations which result in different responses to medications. Beta-2 adrenergic receptor polymorphisms have been associated with beta-receptor sub-sensitization if beta-2 agonists are administered continuously in the absence of cortico-steroids, leading to increased BHR and deteriorating asthma control. Polymorphisms in the 5-lipoxigenase genes result in lack of improvement when treated with the leukotriene receptor antagonist, Montelukast. With the advent of personalized medicine, these pharmaco-genetic insights will aid decisions on therapeutic approaches to asthma management [19].

3. Wheeze Phenotypes

Based on longitudinal birth cohort studies, several distinct wheezing phenotypes have been characterized, each of which have different clinical courses [20]. The understanding emerging from studies of gene environment interactions, as outlined above, begin to explain the underlying mechanisms involved with each phenotype (Figure 2). Early life transient and more prolonged pre-school wheezing is related to gene/environment interactions adversely affecting airway form, function and susceptibility to infection. Indeed, infant wheeze is often preceded by airway function deficits detectable at birth and commonly related to maternal pregnancy smoking [21]. The same factors may be associated with adult onset non-allergic asthma and COPD [6]. More persistent wheeze in childhood beyond 3–5 years of age is mostly associated with allergy.

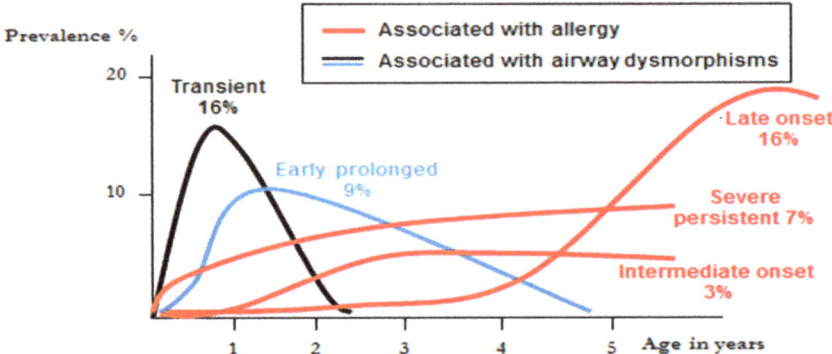

Figure 2. A graphic representation of data from the Avon longitudinal birth cohort study [20], showing the distributions of five wheeze phenotypes over the first five years of life.

4. Early Life Origins of Allergy

Studies of the ontogeny of allergy have increasingly focused on the first 1000 days, from conception to 2 years of age. There is a sequence of events which interact to affect the relative risk of allergy development. The decidual tissues around the fetus promote a Th2 and T-cell regulatory environment through the generation of IL4, IL13, and Transforming Growth Factor beta (TGFβ), which are normal components of the mechanisms generating protection against a maternal Th1 response to fetal–paternal antigens [22]. Absence of this regulation is associated with recurrent early miscarriage and intra-uterine growth retardation, in both murine models and humans [23]. The fetus has the capacity to switch on adaptive immune responses via lymphoid accumulations in the small bowel from the middle of the second trimester of pregnancy [24]. Fetal allergen exposure, in association with Th2-promoting cytokines, occurs via swallowed amniotic fluid in the second trimester, and antigen presentation and sensitization can occur through the fetal gut. Consequently, all neonates have a Th2-biased immune response, which is more entrenched when the mother is also allergic [25]. Balancing of the response occurs in the third trimester, through allergen aggregated with IgG transported across the placenta, which down-regulates sensitization through inhibitory IgG receptors. This has been demonstrated by studies showing strong associations between raised IgG antibodies to both ingestant and inhalant allergens in cord blood, and a lower subsequent risk of allergic sensitization [26,27]. One remarkable observational study showed that children of mothers who had undergone rye-grass allergen immunotherapy during pregnancy, and consequently had high IgG antibody levels, compared to children born to rye-grass allergic mothers not receiving immunotherapy, showed fewer positive allergy skin tests to rye-grass 3–12 years later in the offspring [28].

Likely the most important post-natal influence balancing the immune response is diversification of the neonatal microbiome. This explains the association between Caesarean section delivery, or maternal pregnancy antibiotic exposure, and increased risks of food allergy in the offspring [29,30]. In both circumstances, the infant is not exposed to a normal maternal microbiome, by either avoiding passage through the birth-canal or encountering one modified by the antibiotics. Additional and potentially critical reinforcement of neonatal microbiome diversification is provided by a range of factors, including pre-biotic oligosaccharides in human breast milk [31]. Rapid diversification of the gut microbiome is associated with a lower risk of later allergic disease [32]. The post-natal gut and liver in the presence of a normal microbiome, in the absence of co-stimulatory signals, induce tolerance to swallowed antigens/allergens. Later in infancy, early admission to day care, or having an older sibling, is associated with increased early minor respiratory infections, but reduced later risk of allergic disease. This was the origin of what became known as the "hygiene hypothesis", now better described as the "microbial exposure hypothesis" [33].

5. Prevention and Treatment of Allergy

Based on an understanding of the ontogeny of allergy, it is likely that allergen avoidance will have no role in primary prevention of allergic sensitization. Indeed, several studies both in relation to food and inhalant allergy have indicated that early high exposure, from conception through the first months of life, may reduce the later risk of allergic sensitization and disease. Increased levels of IgG-specific antibodies in cord blood, reflecting high maternal exposure to food and inhalant allergens, are transferred across the placenta from mother to fetus in the last trimester of pregnancy, and are associated with a lower risk of later allergic sensitization in infants [26–28]. There is not a linear relationship between exposure and allergy. There is a bell-shaped curve, with low levels being insufficient to switch on a response, while high levels induce immune tolerance by creating anergy or deletion of sensitized T-lymphocytes. Intermediate exposure is more likely to be associated with sensitization and the evolution of allergic disease [34].

Aero-allergen exposure, in those who have rhinitis and/or asthma and are already allergically sensitized, induces immediate (within minutes) mast-cell degranulation, and thereby sneezing, rhinorrhoea, coughing and wheezing. In those with more severe disease, a late inflammatory reaction, dominated by first neutrophils and then eosinophils, evolves three to four hours later. The immediate response is self-limiting, and can be completely reversed by antihistamines for rhinitis and bronchodilators for asthma, while the late reaction is poorly anti-histamine/bronchodilator responsive and is only abrogated by prior treatment with inhaled (or oral/parenteral) cortico-steroids (ICS). The late reaction occurs more frequently in those with more severe airway disease [34]. This provides a basis for understanding the place of each medication in a therapeutic strategy.

Implicit to the knowledge that allergen exposure aggravates pre-existing allergic airway disease is the concept that allergen avoidance will be of benefit. However, many trials have failed to demonstrate consistent efficacy, particularly in relation to house dust mite (HDM) allergic asthma/rhinitis. This has led to Cochrane systematic reviews, reaching the conclusion that allergen avoidance has no place in therapeutic algorithms [35]. The difficulty is that exposures occur in many places, and strategies to reduce aero-allergen levels, whether to HDM, animals, pollens or molds, have been insufficient. There is evidence that perfect avoidance, such as in high altitude environments, as in the Alps, can have considerable benefits [36]. Furthermore, recent trials of an effective environmental control system, based on temperature controlled laminar airflow, employed overnight, have shown significant improvements in quality of life and eosinophilic airway inflammation (represented by raised exhaled nitric oxide levels) in severe asthma in children and adults [37,38]. While guidelines for asthma management have tended to consider allergen avoidance as secondary to pharmaco-therapy [39], those for rhinitis have given this approach a higher priority [40].

6. The Allergic March

The usual representation of the allergic march presents food allergy, followed in succession by eczema, asthma, and finally hay fever. The implication is that one condition leads inexorably to another. However, as our understanding of the genetic basis of eczema and asthma has increased, it has become clear that there are independent influences on each. Nevertheless, there are mechanistic explanations for progression through the march for a proportion of subjects. The genetic basis for eczema is a defect in skin barrier function, of which the best known is polymorphisms in the gene coding for filaggrin. Defects in this protein lead to increased fluid losses from the epidermis, and greater susceptibility to inflammation induced by irritants and micro-organisms, thereby leading to eczema. The defect also renders the skin more susceptible to allergen penetration into the dermis, where antigen-presenting cells can pick up allergens and migrate to regional lymphoid accumulations for sensitization to occur [41]. Thus, the sequence of the march is incorrect, with food allergy a consequence of the gene defect contributing to eczema, and more likely to follow rather than precede it. Inhalant allergy may also evolve by the same route and increase the risk of rhinitis and asthma, though likely only if there is also airway dysmorphism. This could be viewed as a true march, though it may be better to view the overall allergic diseases' associations as a complex stop/start dance—Figure 3 [42].

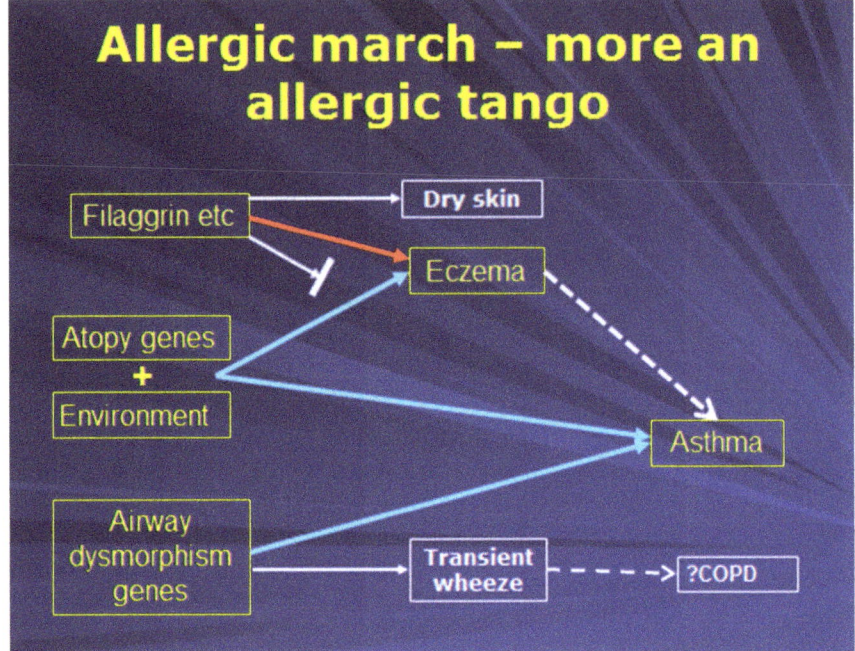

Figure 3. An illustration of the complex relationships between various allergic phenotypes. Constituting not an allergic march but more a complex dance such as the tango.

The other discrepancy in the conventional representation of the march is that rhinitis is more likely to precede rather than follow the development of asthma. This is very clear in the evolution of occupational allergic airway disease. Sensitization to the occupational allergen is followed by rhinitis and skin manifestations. Asthma develops after more sustained exposures. Provided avoidance is instituted early, asthma can be prevented or completely resolved. However, if exposure continues, eventually asthma becomes entrenched and will continue even if the occupational allergen is avoided [43]. If this sequence occurs in allergic asthma, as is very likely, then early avoidance of the primary allergic trigger could have much greater benefit than has been achieved once asthma has reached a chronic stage, with structural (remodeling) changes to the airway wall. This approach requires more research trials.

7. Pharmaco-Therapy for United Airway Diseases

The nose should be considered as the most accessible segment of the respiratory tract. The epithelial lining is identical throughout the conducting airways, and the histo-pathology of allergic inflammation is very similar. From a German longitudinal study, amongst those with allergic rhinitis before 5 years of age, the relative risk for asthma from 5–13 years of age is increased at 3.82%, and 41.5% of children aged 5–13 with new onset wheezing had preceding allergic rhinitis [44]. Conversely, allergic rhinitis co-exists in at least 85% of those with asthma, but is commonly not detected. Perhaps more importantly, treatment of the rhinitis significantly improves asthma control [45].

Mild intermittent airway disease can be treated with non-sedating antihistamines for rhinitis, and bronchodilators as necessary for wheeze. Persistent disease must be treated with regular ICS to achieve control. For those with poor asthma control, long-acting beta agonists (LABAs) and/or leukotriene receptor antagonists (LtRAs) can be added to ICS [39,40]. For the most severe disease, new pharmacological and biological agents are beginning to gain regulatory approval (see following section).

8. Allergen Immunotherapy

While Cochrane systematic reviews have established that subcutaneous allergen immunotherapy improves both rhinitis and asthma, the potential for life-threatening anaphylactic reactions in those with severe asthma means that, at present, its only recommended use in the UK is for allergic rhinitis and insect venom allergy [46]. Its use in allergic rhinitis is clearly established [40]. Furthermore, there is increasing evidence that this approach to management is the only one which truly modifies the natural history of allergic airway disease. Pollen immunotherapy, administered over three consecutive years, had a prolonged carry-over effect for several years after stopping treatment [47]. Furthermore, allergen immunotherapy for three years in children with allergic rhinitis alone reduced the subsequent risk of developing new allergies and asthma [48,49]. The advent of sub-lingual and epidermal vaccines, and modification of allergens, including immunogenic allergen peptides, is beginning to change practice [50]. These beneficial effects of treatment directly addressing allergy demonstrate that allergy has a major impact on asthma severity as an inciter, even if it is not the cause (inducer) of disease. With increasing evidence of safety and efficacy, it is likely that allergen immunotherapy will be used much more extensively in the future.

9. New Approaches to Management of Allergic Airway Diseases

The very worst allergic airway disease can be improved with monoclonal Anti-IgE, administered by sub-cutaneous injections (Omalizumab) [51]. This is the first biological agent to be approved for use in severe asthma. It binds circulating IgE, thereby preventing its attachment to IgE receptors, which consequently down-regulate with long-term treatment. So far there is no evidence that this therapy modifies long-term outcomes in the same way as allergen immunotherapy. It has also been employed, with benefit, in allergic rhinitis, severe eczema, persistent urticaria, and as an adjunct to allergen immunotherapy, however its high costs preclude use other than in the most severe forms of allergic disease [52].

More recently, monoclonal antibodies have been developed which target Interleukin 5 (IL5) or its receptor, which is a key cytokine in mediating eosinophilic inflammation. Amongst these, Mepolizumab, Reslizumab and Benralizumab have been approved by the National Institute for Health and Clinical Excellence for use in severe eosinophilic asthma [53].

Mono-clonal antibodies have been developed which block the activity of IL 4 and 13, which are key cytokines inducing much of the pathology of allergic disease. One such product, Dupilumab, blocks the alpha sub-unit of the IL4 receptor, thereby inhibiting the effects of both IL4 and IL13. It has been shown to improve severe asthma and eczema [54].

Prostaglandin D2 receptors on Th2 lymphocytes mediate much of the allergic inflammatory response. Fevipiprant is an orally active inhibitor of this receptor, which has had variable beneficial effects for eczema and asthma [54].

These new developments make understanding of basic mechanisms an imperative to utilizing novel biological agents, personalized to what has become known as the patient's endo-type (combination of clinical and immunological characteristics).

10. A Shared Misunderstanding between Patient and Physician

The most important component of management is the development of an accord between physician, patient and carer, to achieve concordance with the treatment plan. Patients and carers have first-hand experience of the triggers of exacerbations of airway symptoms. They expect that clinicians will aid identification and confirmation that such triggers are relevant. While it is incumbent on clinicians to address the concerns of their patients, many do not believe that testing for allergic triggers is either necessary or likely to make a difference to treatment. This is often based on the negative Cochrane review of HDM avoidance. The failure to even consider the patient's perception of their disease is likely to lead to a mutual misunderstanding, where an accord has not been reached and concordance with therapeutic recommendations will not be achieved [55]. Furthermore, allergy, to foods and inhalant allergens, is a common association with life-threatening and fatal asthma. Lack of attention to allergic triggers will therefore not only affect concordance but could have severe adverse consequences. My view is that all patients with rhinitis and asthma should have a full allergy-focused history and should be tested for relevant allergy triggers.

Patient/carer education and training, particularly in the use of inhaler devices and monitoring of disease control, is imperative. There must be clear guidance on how to recognize loss of disease control and what action to take. A written, personalized, mutually agreed asthma action plan must be formulated to aid on-going treatment and provide a strategy in event of deterioration in control. Any exacerbation must be considered a failure of control, with the need for immediate review to establish the cause and adjust management accordingly [56].

11. Conclusions

Asthma and rhinitis are commonly associated with allergy, particularly in younger age groups. While allergy and subsequent allergen exposure exacerbates pre-existing airway disease, it is unclear to what extent allergic sensitization is a disease-inducer. Recent insights into the gene-environment interactions suggest that there are often independent influences on allergy and airway disease susceptibility. In some circumstances, changes in airway morphology precede the development and may even facilitate allergic sensitization. In other cases, allergy causes changes in airway morphology, leading to rhinitis and asthma, most obviously with occupational allergen exposures. Therefore, the analogy of which comes first—the chicken or egg—is a circuitous argument. Nevertheless, understanding the early life origins and basic mechanisms will aid the employment of the most appropriate management strategies. Evidence suggests that allergen avoidance to prevent allergic sensitization, which constitutes primary prevention, is ineffective and based on immunological insights is an inappropriate strategy. However, addressing allergy either by avoidance or allergen immunotherapy is an important component of management of those already allergically sensitized, and can be viewed as secondary prevention. Clinicians ignoring any one component of the triad (rhinitis, asthma and allergy) do so at their own, and their patients', peril.

Conflicts of Interest: The author declares no conflict of interest.

References

1. Sunyer, J.; Jarvis, D.; Pekkanen, J.; Chinn, S.; Janson, C.; Leynaert, B.; Luczynska, C.; Garcia-Esteban, R.; Burney, P.; Antó, J.M.; et al. Geographic variations in the effect of atopy on asthma in the European Community Respiratory Health Study. *J. Allergy Clin. Immunol.* **2004**, *114*, 1033–1039. [CrossRef] [PubMed]
2. Warner, J.O.; Boner, A.L. Paediatric Allergy and Asthma. In *Allergy*, 4th ed.; Holgate, S.T., Church, M.K., Broide, D.H., Martinez, F.D., Eds.; Elsevier: Amsterdam, The Netherlands, 2012; pp. 347–360.
3. Collins, S.A.; Lockett, G.A.; Holloway, J.W. The genetics of allergic diseases and asthma. In *Pediatric Allergy Principles and Practice*, 3rd ed.; Leung, Y.M., Sampson, H.A., Geha, R.S., Szefler, S.J., Eds.; Elsevier: Amsterdam, The Netherlands, 2016; pp. 18–30.
4. Van Eerdewegh, P.; Little, R.D.; Dupuis, J.; Del Mastro, R.G.; Falls, K.; Simon, J.; Torrey, D.; Pandit, S.; McKenny, J.; Braunschweiger, K.; et al. Association of the ADAM33 gene with asthma and bronchial hyper-responsiveness. *Nature* **2002**, *418*, 426–443. [CrossRef] [PubMed]
5. Moffatt, M.F.; Kabesch, M.; Liang, L.; Dixon, A.L.; Strachan, D.; Heath, S.; Depner, M.; von Berg, A.; Bufe, A.; Rietschel, E.; et al. Genetic variants regulating ORMDL3 expression contribute to the risk of childhood asthma. *Nature* **2007**, *448*, 470–473. [CrossRef] [PubMed]

6. Davies, E.R.; Kelly, J.F.C.; Howarth, P.H.; Wilson, D.I.; Holgate, S.T.; Davies, D.E.; Whitsett, J.A.; Haitchicorresponding, H.M. Soluble ADAM33 initiates airway remodeling to promote susceptibility for allergic asthma in early life. *JCI Insight.* **2016**, *1*, e87632. [CrossRef] [PubMed]
7. Torgerson, D.G.; Ampleford, E.J.; Chiu, G.Y.; Gauderman, W.J.; Gignoux, C.R.; Graves, P.E.; Himes, B.E.; Levin, A.M.; Mathias, R.A.; Hancock, D.B.; et al. Meta-analysis of Genome-wide Association Studies of Asthma In Ethnically Diverse North American Populations. *Nat. Genet.* **2011**, *43*, 887–892.
8. Moffatt, M.F.; Gut, I.G.; Demenais, F.; Strachan, D.P.; Bouzigon, E.; Heath, S.; von Mutius, E.; Farrall, M.; Lathrop, M.; Cookson, W.O.C.M.; et al. A Large-Scale, Consortium-Based Genome wide Association Study of Asthma. *N. Engl. J. Med.* **2010**, *363*, 1211–1221. [CrossRef]
9. Lee, Y.-L.; Lin, Y.C.; Lee, Y.C.; Wang, J.Y.; Hsiue, T.R.; Guo, Y.L. Glutathione S-transferase P1 gene polymorphism and air pollution as interactive risk factors for childhood asthma. *Clin. Exp. Allergy* **2004**, *334*, 1707–1713. [CrossRef]
10. Eyers, S.; Weatherall, M.; Jefferies, S.; Beasley, R. Paracetamol in pregnancy and the risk of wheezing in offspring: A systematic review and meta-analysis. *Clin. Exp. Allergy* **2011**, *41*, 482–489. [CrossRef]
11. Beasley, R.; Clayton, T.; Crane, J.; von Mutius, E.; Lai, C.K.; Montefort, S.; Stewart, A.; ISAAC Phase Three Study Group. Association between paracetamol use in infancy and childhood, and risk of asthma, rhinoconjunctivitis, and eczema in children aged 6–7 years: Analysis from Phase Three of the ISAAC programme. *Lancet* **2008**, *372*, 1039–1048. [CrossRef]
12. Perzanowski, M.S.; Miller, R.L.; Tang, D.; Ali, D.; Garfinkel, R.S.; Chew, G.L.; Goldstein, I.F.; Perera, F.P.; Barr, R.G. Prenatal acetaminophen exposure and risk of wheeze at age 5 years in an urban low-income cohort. *Thorax* **2010**, *65*, 118–123. [CrossRef]
13. Bønnelykke, K.; Sparks, R.; Waage, J.; Milner, J.D. Genetics of allergy and allergic sensitization: Common variants, rare mutations. *Curr. Opin. Immunol.* **2015**, *36*, 115–126. [CrossRef] [PubMed]
14. Yokouchi, Y.; Nukaga, Y.; Shibasaki, M.; Noguchi, E.; Kimura, K.; Ito, S.; Nishihara, M.; Yamakawa-Kobayashi, K.; Takeda, K.; Imoto, N.; et al. Significant evidence for linkage of mite-sensitive childhood asthma to chromosome 5q31-q33 near the interleukin 12 B locus by a genome-wide search in Japanese families. *Genomics* **2000**, *66*, 152–160. [CrossRef] [PubMed]
15. Xu, C.-J.; Söderhäll, C.; Bustamante, M.; Baïz, N.; Gruzieva, O.; Gehring, U.; Mason, D.; Chatzi, L.; Basterrechea, M.; Llop, S.; et al. DNA methylation in childhood asthma: An epigenome-wide meta-analysis. *Lancet Respir. Med.* **2018**, *6*, 379–388. [CrossRef]
16. Munthe-Kaas, M.C.; Willemse, B.W.M.; Koppelman, G.H. Genetics and epigenetics of childhood asthma. *Eur. Respir. Monogr.* **2012**, *56*, 97–114.
17. Lodge, C.J.; Brabak, L.; Lowe, A.J.; Dharmage, S.C.; Olsson, D.; Forsberg, B. Grandmaternal smoking increases asthma risk in grandchildren: A nationwide Swedish cohort. *Clin. Exp. Allergy* **2018**, *48*, 167–174. [CrossRef]
18. Veeranki, S.P.; Gebretsadik, T.; Mitchel, E.F.; Tylavsky, F.A.; Hartert, T.V.; Cooper, W.O.; Dupont, W.D.; Dorris, S.L.; Hartman, T.J.; Carroll, K.N. Maternal Folic Acid Supplementation during Pregnancy and Early Childhood Asthma. *Epidemiology* **2015**, *26*, 934–941. [CrossRef]
19. Kazani, S.; Wechsler, M.E.; Israel, E. The role of pharmacogenetics in improving the management of asthma. *J. Allergy Clin. Immunol.* **2010**, *125*, 295–302. [CrossRef]
20. Henderson, J.; Granell, R.; Heron, J.; Sherriff, A.; Simpson, A.; Woodcock, A.; Strachan, D.P.; Shaheen, S.O.; Sterne, J.A. Associations of wheezing phenotypes in the first 6 years of life with atopy, lung function and airway responsiveness in mid-childhood. *Thorax* **2008**, *63*, 974–980. [CrossRef]
21. Bisgaard, H.; Loland, L.; Holst, K.K.; Pipper, C.B. Prenatal determinants of neonatal lung function in high-risk newborns. *J. Allergy Clin. Immunol.* **2009**, *123*, 651–657. [CrossRef]
22. Warner, J.O. The early life origins of asthma and related allergic disorders. *Arch. Dis. Child* **2004**, *89*, 97–102. [CrossRef]
23. Warner, J.O. Developmental origins of asthma and related allergic disorders. In *Developmental Origins of Health and Disease*; Gluckman, P., Hanson, M., Eds.; Cambridge Univ. Press: Cambridge, UK, 2006; pp. 349–369.
24. Jones, C.A.; Warner, J.A.; Warner, J.O. Fetal swallowing of IgE. *Lancet* **1998**, *351*, 1859. [CrossRef]
25. Jones, C.A.; Vance, G.H.S.; Power, L.L.; Pender, S.L.F.; MacDonald, T.T.; Warner, J.O. Costimulatory molecules in the developing human gastrointestinal tract: A pathway for fetal allergen priming. *J. Allergy Clin. Immunol.* **2001**, *108*, 235–241. [CrossRef] [PubMed]

26. Jenmalm, M.C.; Björksten, B. Cord blood levels of immune-globulin-G subclass antibodies to food and inhalant allergens in relation to maternal atopy and the development of atopic disease during the first 8 years of life. *Clin. Exp. Allergy* **2000**, *30*, 34–40. [CrossRef] [PubMed]
27. Vance, G.H.S.; Grimshaw, K.E.C.; Briggs, R.; Lewis, S.A.; Mullee, M.A.; Thornton, C.A.; Warner, J.O. Serum ovalbumin-specific immunoglobulinG responses during pregnancy reflect maternal intake of dietary egg and relate to the development of allergy in early infancy. *Clin. Exp. Allergy* **2004**, *34*, 1855–1861. [CrossRef]
28. Glovsky, M.M.; Ghekiere, L.; Rejzek, E. Effect of maternal immunotherapy on immediate skin test reactivity, specific Rye-1 IgG & IgE antibody and total IgE of the children. *Ann. Allergy* **1991**, *67*, 21–24.
29. Mitselou, N.; Hallberg, J.; Stephansson, O.; Almqvist, C.; Melén, E.; Ludvigsson, J.F. Cesarean delivery, preterm birth, and risk of food allergy: Nationwide Swedish cohort study of more than 1 million children. *J. Allergy Clin. Immunol.* **2018**, *142*, 1510–1514.e2. [CrossRef]
30. Hirsch, A.G.; Pollak, J.; Glass, T.A.; Poulsen, M.N.; Bailey-Davis, L.; Mowery, J.; Schwartz, B.S. Early-life antibiotic use and subsequent diagnosis of food allergy and allergic diseases. *Clin. Exp. Allergy* **2017**, *47*, 236–244. [CrossRef]
31. van den Elsen, L.W.J.; Garssen, J.; Burcelin, R.; Verhasselt, V. Shaping the Gut Microbiota by Breastfeeding: The Gateway to Allergy Prevention? *Front. Pediatr.* **2019**, *7*, 47. [CrossRef]
32. Harm Wopereis, H.; Kathleen Sim, K.; Alexander Shaw, A.; Warner, J.O.; Knol, J.; Kroll, J.S. Intestinal microbiota in infants at high risk for allergy: Effects of prebiotics and role in eczema developmentin high risk newborns. *J. Allergy Clin. Immunol.* **2018**, *141*, 1334–1348. [CrossRef]
33. Holt, P.; Naspitz, C.; Warner, J.O. Early immunological influences in prevention of allergy and allergic disease. *Chem. Immunol. Allergy* **2004**, *84*, 102–127.
34. Warner, J.O.; Turner, P.J. *Allergy*; The Science of Paediatrics; Lissauer, T., Carroll, W., Eds.; Elsevier: Amsterdam, The Netherlands, 2017; pp. 297–316.
35. Gøtzsche, P.C.; Johansen, H.K. House dust mite control measures for asthma. *Cochrane Database Syst. Rev.* **2008**, CD001187. [CrossRef] [PubMed]
36. Peroni, D.G.; Boner, A.L.; Vallone, G.; Antolini, I.; Warner, J.O. Effective allergen avoidance at high altitude reduces allergen induced bronchial hyperresponsiveness. *Am. J. Respir. Crit. Care Med.* **1994**, *149*, 1442–1446. [CrossRef] [PubMed]
37. Boyle, R.J.; Pedroletti, C.; Wickman, M.; Bjermer, L.; Valovirta, E.; Dahl, R.; von Berg, A.; Zetterström, O.; Warner, J.O.; for the 4A Study Group. Nocturnal temperature controlled laminar airflow for treating atopic asthma: A randomised controlled trial. *Thorax* **2012**, *67*, 215–221. [CrossRef]
38. Warner, J.O. Use of temperature-controlled laminar airflow in the management of atopic asthma: Clinical evidence and experience. *Adv. Respir. Dis.* **2017**, *11*, 181–188. [CrossRef]
39. British Thoracic Society/Scottish Intercollegiate Guidelines Network. *British Guideline on the Management of Asthma*; British Thoracic Society: London, UK, 2016.
40. Brożek, J.L.; Bousquet, J.; Baena-Cagnani, C.E.; Bonini, S.; Canonica, G.W.; Casale, T.B.; van Wijk, R.G.; Ohta, K.; Zuberbier, T.; Schünemann, H.J.; et al. Allergic Rhinitis and its Impact on Asthma (ARIA) guidelines: 2010 revision. *J. Allergy Clin. Immunol.* **2010**, *126*, 466–476. [CrossRef]
41. McLean, W.H.I. Filaggrin failure—From ichthyosis vulgaris to atopic eczema and beyond. *Brit. J. Derm.* **2016**, *175*, 4–7. [CrossRef]
42. Levin, M.E.; Warner, J.O. The Atopic Dance. *Curr. Allergy Clin. Immunol.* **2017**, *30*, 146–149.
43. Moscato, G. Occupational allergic airway disease. *Curr. Otorhinolaryngol. Rep.* **2017**, *5*, 220. [CrossRef]
44. Rochat, M.K.; Illi, S.; Ege, M.J.; Lau, S.; Keil, T.; Wahn, U.; von Mutius, E.; Multicentre Allergy Study (MAS) Group. Allergic rhinitis as a predictor for wheezing onset in school-aged children. *J. Allergy Clin. Immunol.* **2010**, *126*, 1170–1175. [CrossRef]
45. Welsh, P.W.; Stricker, W.E.; Chu, C.-P.; Naessens, J.M.; Naessens, J.M.; Reese, M.E.; Reed, C.E.; Marcoux, J.P. Efficacy of Beclomethasone Nasal Solution, Flunisolide, and Cromolyn in Relieving Symptoms of Ragweed Allergy. *Mayo Clin. Proc.* **1987**, *62*, 125–134. [CrossRef]
46. Abramson, M.J.; Puy, R.M.; Weiner, J.M. Injection allergen immunotherapy for asthma. *Cochrane Database Syst. Rev.* **2010**, CD001186. [CrossRef]
47. Durham, S.R.; Walker, S.M.; Varga, E.-M.; Jacobson, M.R.; O'Brien, F.; Noble, W.; Till, S.J.; Hamid, Q.A.; Nouri-Aria, K.T. Long-Term Clinical Efficacy of Grass-Pollen Immunotherapy. *N. Engl. J. Med.* **1999**, *341*, 468–475. [CrossRef] [PubMed]

48. Eng, P.A.; Borer-Reinhold, M.; Heijnen, I.A.; Gnehm, H.P. Twelve-year follow-up after discontinuation of preseasonal grasspollen immunotherapy in childhood. *Allergy* **2006**, *61*, 198–201. [CrossRef] [PubMed]
49. Jacobsen, L.; Niggemann, B.; Dreborg, S.; Ferdousi, H.A.; Reese, M.E.; Reed, C.E.; Marcoux, J.P. Specific immunotherapy has long-term preventive effect of seasonaland perennial asthma: 10-year follow-up on the PAT study. *Allergy* **2007**, *62*, 943–948. [CrossRef] [PubMed]
50. Pfaar, O.; Lou, H.; Zhang, Y.; Klimek, L.; Zhang, L. Recent developments and highlights in allergen immunotherapy. *Allergy* **2018**. [CrossRef] [PubMed]
51. Incorvaia, C.; Mauro, M.; Makri, E.; Leo, G.; Ridolo, E. Two decades with omalizumab: What we still have to learn. *Biol. Targets Ther.* **2018**, *12*, 135–142. [CrossRef]
52. Warner, J.O. Omalizumab for childhood asthma. *Expert Rev. Resp. Med.* **2010**, *4*, 5–7. [CrossRef]
53. National Institute for Health and Clinical Excellence. *Benralizumab for Treating for Treating Severe Eosinophilic Asthma Eosinophilic*; Technology Appraisal Guidance; National Institute for Health and Clinical Excellence: London, UK, 2019; Available online: nice.org.uk/guidance/ta565 (accessed on 21 April 2020).
54. Abrams, E.M.; Becker, A.B.; Szefler, S.J. Current State and Future of Biologic Therapies in the Treatment of Asthma in Children. *Pediatr. Allergy Immunol. Pulmonol.* **2018**, *31*, 119–131. [CrossRef]
55. Gore, C.; Griffin, R.; Rothenberg, T.; Tallett, A.; Hopwood, B.; Sizmur, S.; O'Keeffe, C.; Warner, J.O. New patient-reported experience measure for children with allergic disease: Development, validation and results from integrated care. *Arch. Dis. Child.* **2016**, *101*, 935–943. [CrossRef]
56. Warner, J.O.; Spitters, S. Integrating Care for Children with Allergic Diseases: UK experience. *Curr. Allergy Clin. Immunol.* **2017**, *30*, 130–135.

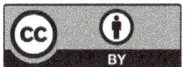

© 2020 by the author. Licensee MDPI, Basel, Switzerland. This article is an open access article distributed under the terms and conditions of the Creative Commons Attribution (CC BY) license (http://creativecommons.org/licenses/by/4.0/).

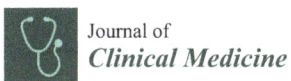

Communication

Global Asthma Network Phase I Surveillance: Geographical Coverage and Response Rates

Philippa Ellwood [1,*], Eamon Ellwood [1], Charlotte Rutter [2], Virginia Perez-Fernandez [3], Eva Morales [4], Luis García-Marcos [3], Neil Pearce [2,5], M Innes Asher [1], David Strachan [6] and on behalf of the GAN Phase I Study Group [†]

1. Department of Paediatrics: Child and Youth Health, Faculty of Medical and Health Sciences, University of Auckland, 1023 Auckland, New Zealand; e.ellwood@auckland.ac.nz (E.E.); i.asher@auckland.ac.nz (M.I.A.)
2. Department of Medical Statistics, London School of Hygiene and Tropical Medicine, London WC1E 7HT, UK; Charlotte.Rutter1@lshtm.ac.uk (C.R.); Neil.Pearce@lshtm.ac.uk (N.P.)
3. Pediatric Allergy and Pulmonology Units, 'Virgen de la Arrixaca' University Children's Hospital, University of Murcia, ARADyAL network and Biomedical Research Institute of Murcia (IMIB-Arrixaca), 30394 Murcia, Spain; virperez@um.es (V.P.-F.); lgmarcos@um.es (L.G.-M.)
4. Biomedical Research Institute of Murcia (IMIB-Arrixaca) and Department of Public Health Sciences, University of Murcia, 30394 Murcia, Spain; embarto@hotmail.com
5. Centre for Global NCDs, London School of Hygiene and Tropical Medicine, London WC1E 7HT, UK
6. Population Health Research Institute, St George's University of London, London SW17 0RE, UK; d.strachan@sgul.ac.uk
* Correspondence: p.ellwood@auckland.ac.nz
† The GAN Phase I Study Group is listed at the end of the manuscript.

Received: 24 September 2020; Accepted: 13 November 2020; Published: 17 November 2020

Abstract: Background—The Global Asthma Network (GAN) Phase I is surveying school pupils in high-income and low- or middle-income countries using the International Study of Asthma and Allergies in Childhood (ISAAC) methodology. Methods—Cross-sectional surveys of participants in two age groups in randomly selected schools within each centre (2015–2020). The compulsory age group is 13–14 years (adolescents), optionally including parents or guardians. Six to seven years (children) and their parents are also optional. Adolescents completed questionnaires at school, and took home adult questionnaires for parent/guardian completion. Children took home questionnaires for parent/guardian completion about the child and also adult questionnaires. Questions related to symptoms and risk factors for asthma and allergy, asthma management, school/work absence and hospitalisation. Results—53 centres in 20 countries completed quality checks by 31 May 2020. These included 21 centres that previously participated in ISAAC. There were 132,748 adolescents (average response rate 88.8%), 91,802 children (average response rate 79.1%), and 177,622 adults, with >97% answering risk factor questions and >98% answering questions on asthma management, school/work absence and hospitalisation. Conclusion—The high response rates achieved in ISAAC have generally been maintained in GAN. GAN Phase I surveys, partially overlapping with ISAAC centres, will allow within-centre analyses of time-trends in prevalence.

Keywords: global; asthma; surveillance; responses; children; adults' epidemiology

1. Introduction

The Global Asthma Network (GAN) [1,2] was formed in 2012 as a joint initiative by members of the International Study of Asthma and Allergies in Childhood (ISAAC) and the International Union Against Tuberculosis and Lung Disease, following their co-production of the first Global Asthma Report (GAR), launched in 2011 at the time of the United Nations high-level meeting on non-communicable diseases [3]. Estimates of the worldwide burden of asthma in that report were based very largely on the

ISAAC Phase III surveys (2001–2003) of 13–14-year-olds (adolescents) and 6–7-year-olds (children) [4], with time trends from centres which also participated in ISAAC Phase I (1994–1995) [5], plus the World Health Surveys of adults (2002–2003) [6]. The need for updated surveillance of asthma prevalence, severity, diagnosis and management, highlighted in GAR 2011 [3], has become more pressing since then [7], as very few studies anywhere in the world have evaluated trends in asthma prevalence and related risk factors over the last decade [8].

GAN Phase I was developed to address this information gap, with these hypotheses:

(1) Globally, the burden of asthma is changing in adults and children;
(2) There is large variation in the diagnosis of asthma;
(3) In many locations, asthma is under-diagnosed and its management is suboptimal; and
(4) There are potentially modifiable risk factors for asthma.

Its aims were:

(1) To conduct asthma surveillance around the world in two age groups of school pupils, and their parents, measuring prevalence, severity, management and risk factors, following the methods of ISAAC Phase III;
(2) To examine time trends in prevalence, severity, management and risk factors from centres which completed ISAAC Phase III; and
(3) To evaluate the appropriateness of asthma management, especially access to quality-assured essential asthma medicines, as defined by WHO [9].

Although modelled closely on the study design and methodology of ISAAC Phase III, GAN Phase I has extended its scope to include adults, for whom there are limited global data on asthma prevalence [8], severity and risk factors, and to assess asthma management, which is commonly suboptimal in low-income settings [7]. This paper summarises the progress of GAN Phase I at 31 May 2020, when the dataset was temporarily frozen for the first round of analyses including centres which completed the quality checks by this date.

2. Methods

GAN has collaborators from 383 centres in 137 countries all of whom answered the call for an Expression of Interest (EOI). Of the EOIs, 136 centres in 58 countries registered to participate in GAN Phase I. Of these registered centres some have completed GAN Phase I and provided data to this study, while some, because of timing, will be included in later publications. Other centres have been unable to undertake Phase I at all because of unforeseen circumstances. Many centres in each of these categories have contributed to other published GAN surveys [10–13].

GAN Phase I is a cross-sectional, multi-centre, multi-country study undertaken between 2015–2020. Its methodology has been described and justified elsewhere [2] and detailed in an online manual [14]. Each centre was required to obtain approval from their local ethics committee prior to the start of their study.

Briefly, each GAN centre is based on a defined geographical area, within which a minimum of 10 schools were selected at random (or all schools, if less than ten). All students of a specified age within these schools were studied, selected by grade/level/year, or by chronological age. The sample size estimates of 1000–3000 are stringent because of the number of hypotheses being tested, and high response rates are sought. As in ISAAC, two age groups of school pupils participated: adolescents and children. Centres that undertook ISAAC Phase III and/or ISAAC Phase I were expected to use the same study design and sampling frame in GAN. As in ISAAC Phase III, translations into the local language were required and centres followed the ISAAC protocol for translation, back translation to English, and comparison between the two [15].

The compulsory age group was adolescents, who self-completed written questionnaires at school. Additionally, in some centres, the ISAAC international video questionnaire showing different scenes of asthma in children of a variety of ethnicities was shown [16]. A self-completed risk factor questionnaire, developed for ISAAC Phase III, was strongly recommended in this age group. In ISAAC surveys, there was no contact with the parents of the adolescent age group, but for GAN, it was recommended (but not essential) that the parents/guardians of the adolescents were also surveyed.

This optional parental questionnaire obtained information on the prevalence of asthma, rhinitis and eczema symptoms among adults, plus questions on asthma management and risk factors. The adult symptoms questionnaire combined items from ISAAC and the European Community Respiratory Health Survey (ECRHS) [17] to cover the range of chest symptoms and diagnoses that might be related to asthma in young and middle-aged adults.

The inclusion of children was optional, as with ISAAC Phase III, who took written questionnaires home to be completed by their parents. These included the ISAAC questionnaire on the child's symptoms used in Phases I and III, and the risk factor questionnaire used in Phase III. In GAN it was recommended (but not essential) to add the parental questionnaire to ascertain the prevalence of asthma, rhinitis and eczema symptoms among adults in the household.

Data from each centre were submitted to the GAN Global Centre (Auckland, New Zealand) together with a descriptive centre report. Following initial quality control checks in Auckland, the data were transferred to one of two designated GAN Phase I data centres for checking and analysis: Murcia (Spain) for Spanish- and Portuguese-speaking centres, and London (United Kingdom), for centres using all other languages. A harmonised approach to data processing, checking and analysis was developed, using Stata versions 13–15.

Estimation of participation rates among children and adolescents followed the conventions previously adopted in ISAAC Phase III. High levels of participation are sought as it is a concern that absent school pupils may be away from school due to symptoms of asthma, rhinitis or eczema. A participation rate of at least 80% for the adolescents and 70% for the children is desirable [2,14]. The denominator was the number of pupils in the cluster sample and the numerator was the number of core symptom questionnaires returned with at least some symptom data.

We were unable to calculate a conventional response rate for the adults as it was not known how many adults received questionnaires (because some schoolchildren have only one parent or guardian). Therefore, a "per child" approach was taken to estimate adult response rate, as follows. The denominator was the number of school-aged respondents (index schoolchildren) to whom one or more adult questionnaires were distributed. The numerator was the number of index schoolchildren for whom one or more adult questionnaires were returned. For centres which distributed adult questionnaires to both age groups of schoolchildren, the numerators and denominators were combined to derive a single estimate of "per child" adult response rate.

It was not possible to derive this measure of adult response rate for three centres (Costa Rica (whole country study), Guatemala City, Guatemala; Tegucigalpa, Honduras) where adult responses were not linked to the child identifier.

3. Results

By 31 May 2020, 53 centres in 20 countries had submitted and completed quality checks of data and methodology. Figure 1 shows the location of these centres, also 84 centres in 38 countries which formally registered an intention to complete GAN Phase I but were unable to do so, and the remaining GAN collaborating centres. Most centres completed their fieldwork before the onset of the COVID-19 pandemic, but surveys were still active in Iran (Yazd and Karaj) and Greece (Athens) in spring 2020, where fieldwork was truncated due to school closures in the pandemic lockdown.

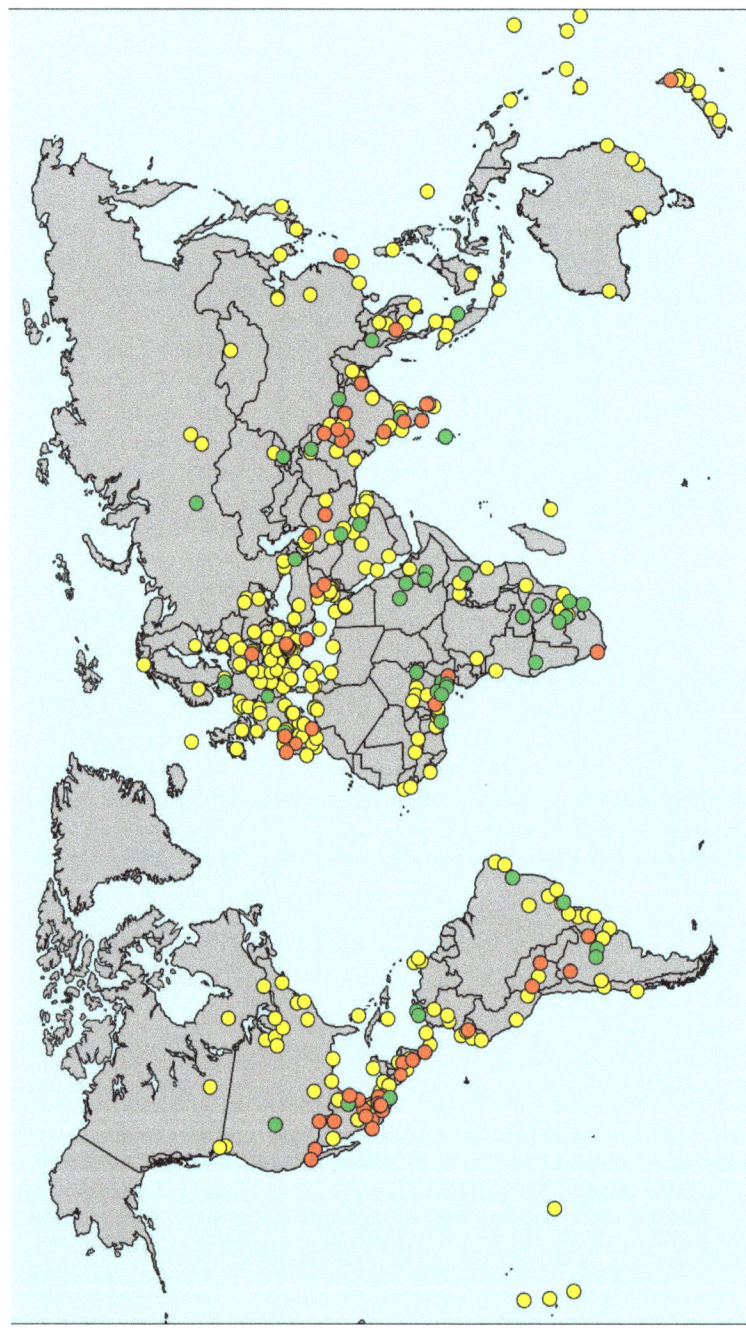

Figure 1. Global Asthma Network (GAN) Centres. Centres registered with GAN identifying those that completed data collection before end of May 2020 (red); registered centres expected to complete GAN Phase I later (green); centres collaborating with GAN but not expected to contribute Phase I data (yellow).

Twenty-one of the 53 centres had previously participated in ISAAC Phase III (including 17 contributing data on both age groups) and 12 had previously participated in ISAAC Phase I (including 9 with data on both age groups). All of the 12 ISAAC Phase I centres except for Athens also participated in ISAAC Phase III. The geographical overlap between ISAAC and GAN centres is shown in Figure 2. Forty of the 53 GAN centres also contributed data on adult symptoms, risk factors and disease management, as summarised in Table 1.

Table 2 summarises the numbers of pupils and number of schools for which responses were received in GAN Phase I, by age group and questionnaire section (symptoms, risk factors, management and morbidity). When deriving the number of valid responses to the asthma management and asthma-related morbidity questions, respondents who legitimately skipped these sections because they had answered negatively to asthma symptoms were included in the count of responders.

Overall, responses were received for 132,748 adolescents attending 1260 schools (with risk factor information on 99.3% and management/morbidity information on 98.8%) and 91,802 children attending 1506 schools (with risk factor information on 99.3% and management/morbidity information on 99.5%). Additionally, there were responses for 177,622 adults, with risk factor information on 97.7% and 98.2% providing information on asthma management, work absence, or hospitalisation. These 177,622 adults relate to 100,011 school pupils that returned adult questionnaires, comprising 50,416 adolescents and 49,595 children.

The stringent response criteria were able to be met by 45 (85%) of the 53 GAN Phase I centres for adolescents, 33 (80%) of the 41 GAN Phase I centres for children and by 24 (65%) of the 37 GAN Phase I centres for adults. Lower rates in some centres occurred due to schools closing because of the COVID-19 pandemic. Table 3 compares the response rates for the core symptom questionnaires by age group for each GAN Phase I centre and the corresponding response rates in earlier ISAAC surveys, where relevant. Across all GAN centres, the mean participation rate was 88.8% for adolescents and 79.1% for children (compared to 88.0% and 84.5%, respectively, in ISAAC Phase III). For GAN Phase I centres which were also ISAAC Phase III centres, mean response rates were 90.0% for adolescents and 79.0% for children in GAN compared with 89.3% and 84.4%, respectively, in ISAAC Phase III. One or more responses to the adult symptom questionnaire were received from an average of 73.2% of households contacted.

Table 1. Number of study centres contributing data for each GAN Phase I module and age-group, with corresponding data for International Study of Asthma and Allergies in Childhood (ISAAC) Phases I and III.

Questionnaire Module	GAN Phase I Centres			ISAAC Phase III Centres *		ISAAC Phase I Centres *	
	6–7	13–14	Adults	6–7	13–14	6–7	13–14
Symptoms:							
Asthma (written)	41	53	40	144 [17]	233 [21]	91 [9]	155 [12]
Asthma (video)	NA	29	NA	NA	139 [8]	NA	99 [3]
Rhinoconjunctivitis	41	53	NA	144 [17]	233 [21]	91 [9]	155 [12]
Eczema	41	53	40	142 [17]	231 [21]	91 [9]	155 [12]
Risk factors:							
ISAAC Phase 3 questions	40	52	38	75 [17]	122 [21]	ND	ND
Active smoking	NA	52	38	ND	ND	ND	ND
Perinatal questions	39	NA	NA	ND	ND	ND	ND
Indoor environment	39	NA	38	ND	ND	ND	ND
Asthma-related:							
Management (now)	41	53	40	ND	ND	ND	ND
Management (infancy)	39	NA	NA	ND	ND	ND	ND
School absence	41	53	40	ND	ND	ND	ND
Work absence	NA	NA	40	ND	ND	ND	ND
Hospitalisation	41	53	40	ND	ND	ND	ND

* Numbers of centres also participating in GAN Phase I in parentheses. NA Not applicable (module not included for that age group). ND No data (module not included in ISAAC data collection).

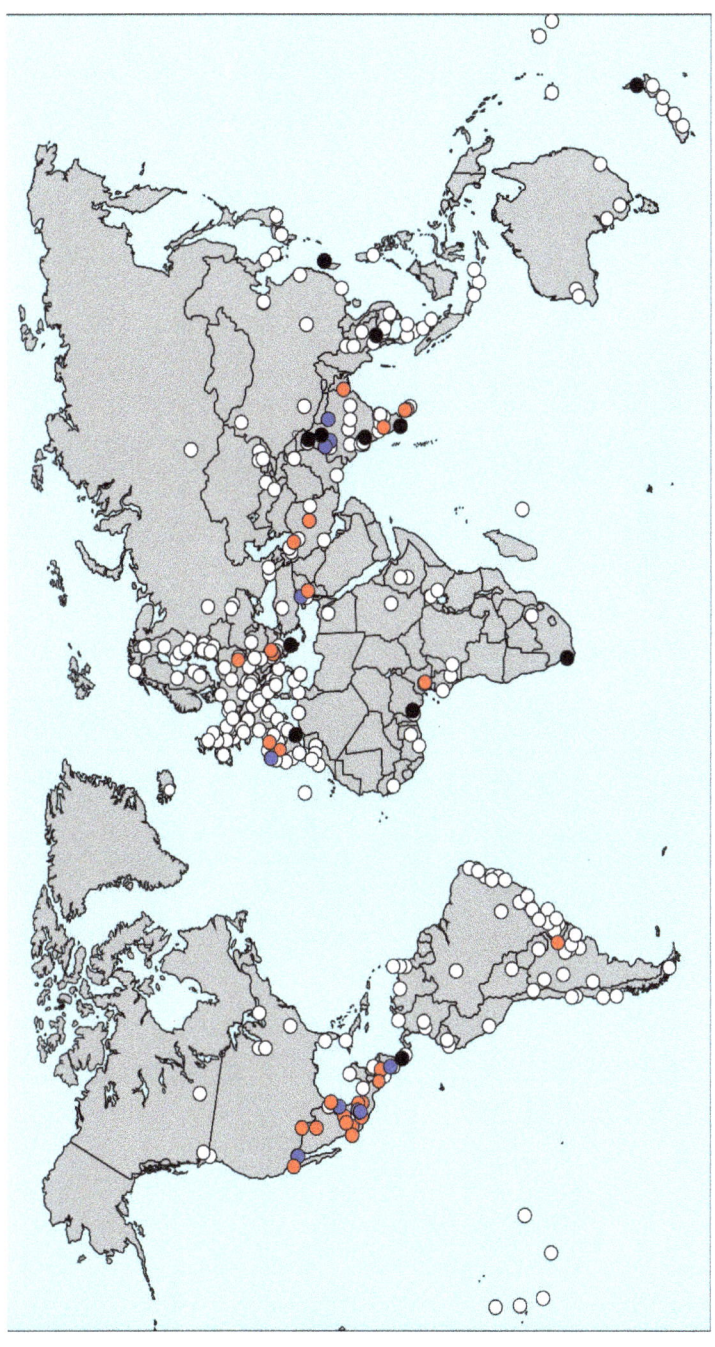

Figure 2. Overlap of GAN Phase I and ISAAC Centres. Centres that completed GAN Phase I checks before 31 May 2020 (red); GAN Phase I centres included in ISAAC Phase III but not ISAAC Phase I (blue); GAN Phase I centres included in ISAAC Phase I and ISAAC Phase III (black*); ISAAC Phase III only centres (white). * Athens, Greece contributed data to GAN and ISAAC Phase I, but not ISAAC Phase III.

Table 2. Number of participants (P) and number of schools (S) responding to each GAN module by study centre and age-group.

Centre Name	6–7-Year-Olds						13–14-Year-Olds						Adults					
	Symptoms		Risk Factors		Management		Symptoms		Risk Factors		Management		Symptoms		Risk Factors		Management	
	P	S	P	S	P	S	P	S	P	S	P	S	P	S	P	S	P	S
Yaounde	722	27	722	27	703	27	1066	22	1066	22	1056	22	860	32	832	32	824	32
Ibadan	0	0	0	0	0	0	2897	23	2894	23	2810	23	2321	23	2321	23	2217	23
Cape Town	0	0	0	0	0	0	3979	29	3976	29	3879	29	0	0	0	0	0	0
Taipei	3036	25	3036	25	3034	25	3474	24	3465	24	3464	24	9689	49	9673	49	9594	49
Bangkok	3067	7	3067	7	3063	7	3206	6	3201	6	3084	6	5418	13	5416	13	5311	13
Yazd	0	0	0	0	0	0	5141	48	5141	48	5141	48	0	0	0	0	0	0
Karaj	572	39	0	0	572	39	754	42	0	0	754	42	1175	75	0	0	1175	75
Lattakia	1115	9	1078	9	1111	9	1215	10	1214	10	1203	10	0	0	0	0	0	0
Damascus	0	0	0	0	0	0	1100	11	1100	11	1100	11	0	0	0	0	0	0
Kottayam	2099	50	2099	50	2085	50	2090	20	2088	20	2050	20	6940	69	6937	69	6743	69
New Delhi	2516	54	2516	54	2516	54	3024	59	3024	59	3024	59	9449	113	9449	113	9010	113
Chandigarh	2473	57	2473	57	2473	57	3000	54	3000	54	2999	54	10,386	111	10,386	111	10,384	111
Bikaner	2600	45	2600	45	2551	45	2702	33	2702	33	2702	33	10,495	78	10,495	78	10,473	78
Jaipur	2296	44	2296	44	2250	44	3060	57	3057	57	2977	57	8933	101	8902	101	8524	101
iLucknow	2969	32	2969	32	2931	32	2968	31	2969	31	2933	31	11,820	63	11,786	63	11,405	63
Kolkata	0	0	0	0	0	0	2998	37	2998	37	2886	37	7823	91	7818	91	7547	91
Pune	2404	26	2404	26	2403	26	3030	34	3030	34	3021	34	8000	60	7994	60	7909	60
Mysuru (Mysore)	2730	30	2730	30	2730	30	3051	29	3051	29	3051	29	11,178	59	11,178	59	11,177	59
Peradeniya	1492	12	1492	12	1455	12	1696	11	1696	11	1547	11	0	0	0	0	0	0
Anuradhapura	2180	10	2180	10	2120	10	2986	10	2989	10	2638	10	0	0	0	0	0	0
Uruguaiana	0	0	0	0	0	0	1058	17	1052	17	1057	17	896	17	896	17	884	17
Costa Rica	1936	34	1936	34	1936	34	1338	33	1338	33	1316	33	3272	67	3272	67	3102	67
Guatemala City	1072	39	1072	39	1071	39	1420	42	1408	42	1400	42	1078	30	1078	30	1055	29
Tegucigalpa	361	22	361	22	359	22	1431	65	1431	65	1415	65	254	10	254	10	252	10
Mexico City North	2515	58	2515	58	2498	58	3375	9	3370	9	3375	9	5231	66	5219	66	5104	66
Guadalajara	2082	21	2082	21	2075	21	2519	13	2518	13	2516	13	489	20	487	20	483	20
Mexicali	2001	37	2001	37	1999	37	2479	20	2464	20	2469	20	2436	41	2427	41	2427	41
Ciudad Victoria	2444	20	2444	20	2439	20	2468	8	2465	8	2467	8	6239	28	6202	28	6149	28
San Luis Potosí	2108	28	2108	28	2108	28	2580	19	2580	19	2579	19	2835	27	2833	27	2801	27
Tijuana	2082	47	2082	47	2072	47	2601	13	2595	13	2577	13	1397	26	1395	26	1376	26
Toluca Urban	2712	21	2712	21	2702	21	2650	6	2642	6	2643	6	6162	27	6122	27	6072	27
Toluca Rural	2975	17	2976	17	2974	17	3122	16	3114	16	3091	16	7587	33	7583	33	7470	33
Chihuahua	1969	33	1969	33	1962	33	2180	7	2103	7	2161	7	0	0	0	0	0	0
Ciudad Juárez	2117	39	2118	39	2114	39	2443	16	2439	16	2426	16	2610	37	2598	37	2601	37

Table 2. Cont.

Centre Name	6–7-Year-Olds								13–14-Year-Olds								Adults						
	Symptoms		Risk Factors		Management				Symptoms		Risk Factors		Management				Symptoms		Risk Factors		Management		
	P	S	P	S	P	S			P	S	P	S	P	S			P	S	P	S	P	S	
Michoácan	2166	39	2166	39	2156	39			2504	14	2502	14	2503	14			2232	39	2232	39	2206	39	
Xalapa	3716	83	3717	83	3712	83			3339	21	3335	21	3327	21			0	0	0	0	0	0	
Córdoba	2746	60	2746	60	2738	60			2991	25	2980	25	2989	25			2839	35	2832	35	2829	35	
Puerto Vallarta	2241	46	2241	46	2238	46			2439	15	2439	15	2428	15			0	0	0	0	0	0	
Aguascalientes	3175	19	3176	19	3165	19			3336	19	3334	19	3331	19			2907	33	2898	33	2861	33	
Matamoros	806	24	806	24	799	24			2892	12	2882	12	2865	12			1315	24	1306	24	1298	24	
Managua	3162	59	3162	59	3127	59			3131	50	3126	50	2973	50			0	0	0	0	0	0	
Prishtina	0	0	0	0	0	0			1054	14	1056	14	1052	14			2006	14	2006	14	1977	14	
Gjakova	0	0	0	0	0	0			676	5	676	5	676	5			1352	5	1352	5	1350	5	
Prizren	0	0	0	0	0	0			1427	10	1427	10	1427	10			2712	10	0		2699	10	
Gjilan	0	0	0	0	0	0			1200	6	1200	6	1200	6			1835	6	1835	6	1834	6	
Ferizaj	0	0	0	0	0	0			890	9	890	9	885	9			1371	9	1372	9	1328	9	
Katowice	1462	36	1462	36	1460	36			3185	29	3184	29	3180	29			2220	35	2219	35	2201	35	
Auckland	1538	22	1538	22	1538	22			1885	7	1885	7	1860	7			3002	29	2994	29	2986	29	
Athens	0	0	0	0	0	0			1934	20	1934	20	1934	20			1897	20	1897	20	1897	20	
Cartagena	3509	61	3509	61	3496	61			3436	26	3430	26	3428	26			6961	60	6956	60	6832	60	
Salamanca	2388	51	2388	51	2387	51			3485	31	3484	31	3481	31			0	0	0	0	0	0	
Cantabria	2841	75	2841	75	2836	75			4381	47	4372	47	4374	47			0	0	0	0	0	0	
A Coruña	3407	48	3407	48	3407	48			3462	26	3461	26	3455	26			0	0	0	0	0	0	
All centres	91,802	1506	91,197	1467	91,365	1506			13,2748	1260	131,777	1218	131,179	1260			177,622	1685	173,452	1600	174,367	1684	

Table 3. Response rates for 6–7 and 13–14 year age groups to the written symptom questionnaires in GAN Phase I, ISAAC Phases I and III, by study centre and age-group. (The adult response rate was estimated on a "per child" basis *).

		GAN Phase I				ISAAC Phase III			ISAAC Phase I		
		Survey	Response (%)			Survey	Response (%)		Survey	Response (%)	
Country	Centre Name	Years	6–7	13–14	Adult *	Years	6–7	13–14	Years	6–7	13–14
Cameroon	Yaounde	2018–19	53.8	99.9	34.6 [a]						
Nigeria	Ibadan	2018	-	85.0	79.5 [c]				1995		76.4
South Africa	Cape Town	2017	-	84.4	[d]				1995		82.8
Taiwan	Taipei	2016–17	76.3	93.0	84.5 [a]	2001–02	96.8	95.9	1995	92.2	93.2
Thailand	Bangkok	2017–18	86.3	97.9	86.1 [a]	2001	72.8	93.8	1995–96	90.8	74.8
Iran	Yazd	2020	-	71.3	[d]						
Iran	Karaj	2019–20	72.0	71.9	88.6 [a]						
Syrian Arab Republic	Lattakia	2019	93.0	99.6	[d]	2001–03	99.1	99.8			
Syrian Arab Republic	Damascus	2018	-	91.7	[d]						
India	Kottayam	2017–18	68.4	85.3	97.5 [a]	2001–03	96.4	98.5	1994–95	78.1	90.7
India	New Delhi	2017–18	80.9	100.0	85.7 [a]	2001–02	82.4	86.7	1994–95	99.2	100
India	Chandigarh	2017–18	100.0	100.0	95.5 [a]	2001–02		99.4	1994–95	94.0	97.4
India	Bikaner	2017–18	86.7	90.1	99.8 [a]	2001		95.4			
India	Jaipur	2017–18	75.8	98.7	84.4 [a]	2001	75.4	87.4			
India	Lucknow	2017	91.3	94.0	99.7 [a]	2001–02	85.7	75.0			
India	Kolkata	2017–18	-	99.9	80.2 [c]						
India	Pune	2017–18	79.8	99.6	81.4 [a]	2001–02	90.4	70.8	1994–95	99.6	99.8
India	Mysuru (Mysore)	2017–18	90.9	99.5	97.4 [a]						
Sri Lanka	Peradeniya	2018	74.6	80.8	[d]						
Sri Lanka	Anuradhapura	2018	72.7	85.4	[d]						
Brazil	Uruguaiana	2016–18	-	88.2	76.7 [c]						
Costa Rica	Costa Rica	2017–18	64.5	66.9	[e]	2001–02	80.9	69.6	1994–95	84.1	91.4
Guatemala	Guatemala City	2018	32.2	40.6	[e]						
Honduras	Tegucigalpa	2017–18	76.5	98.0	[e]						
Mexico	Mexico City North	2015–16	86.7	93.8	55.9 [a]	2002–03	91.6	99.8			
Mexico	Guadalajara	2016	83.3	90.0	12.1 [b]						
Mexico	Mexicali	2015–16	77.0	83.7	32.7 [a]	2002–03	74.3	93.6			
Mexico	Ciudad Victoria	2015–16	81.5	82.3	78.6 [a]	2003	73.1	79.5			
Mexico	San Luis Potosi	2015–16	99.4	97.3	36.7 [a]						
Mexico	Tijuana	2015–16	83.3	86.7	41.4 [b]						
Mexico	Toluca Urban	2015–16	95.7	98.1	65.5 [a]	2002	89.5	86.1			
Mexico	Toluca Rural	2015–16	93.0	94.6	69.1 [a]						

Table 3. Cont.

Country	Centre Name	GAN Phase I				ISAAC Phase III			ISAAC Phase I		
		Survey Years	Response (%)			Survey Years	Response (%)		Survey Years	Response (%)	
			6–7	13–14	Adult *		6–7	13–14		6–7	13–14
Mexico	Chihuahua	2015–16	87.5	87.2	[d]						
Mexico	Ciudad Juárez	2016–17	84.7	88.8	36.7 [a]						
Mexico	Michoacán	2016	90.3	92.7	75.8 [b]						
Mexico	Xalapa	2016–17	92.9	90.2	[d]						
Mexico	Córdoba	2016	91.5	93.5	30.2 [a]						
Mexico	Puerto Vallarta	2015–17	93.4	90.3	[d]						
Mexico	Aguascalientes	2015–16	90.7	95.3	44.0 [a]						
Mexico	Matamoros	2015–17	80.6	93.3	93.7 [b]						
Nicaragua	Managua	2018	87.9	90.5	[d]	2002	96.0	94.5			
Kosovo	Prishtina	2017	-	99.9	99.9 [c]						
Kosovo	Gjakova	2018	-	90.1	100.0 [c]						
Kosovo	Prizren	2017	-	89.0	99.7 [c]						
Kosovo	Gjilan	2017	-	80.0	81.5 [c]						
Kosovo	Ferizaj	2017	-	99.9	85.1 [c]						
Poland	Katowice	2017–18	36.8	79.1	85.6 [b]						
New Zealand	Auckland	2018–19	63.7	85.5	51.3 [a]	2001	84.6	92.3	1992–93	90.2	94.6
Greece	Athens	2020	-	75.5	99.9 [c]				1994–95		87.0
Spain	Cartagena	2015–16	65.9	73.8	61.5 [a]	2001–02	72.3	79.6	1993	68.5	95.1
Spain	Salamanca	2017–18	73.7	95.0	[d]						
Spain	Cantabria	2017–18	56.2	77.4	[d]						
Spain	A Coruña	2018–19	71.0	92.1	[d]	2003	73.8	93.6			

* Adult response rate per child, derived as the percentage of schoolchildren that had one or more adult questionnaires returned, combined across age groups when both age groups were studied: (a) both age groups; (b) 6–7-year-olds only; (c) 13–14-year-olds only; (d) neither age group; (e) adult responses not linked to child identifiers, so no response rate for adults can be derived.

4. Discussion

GAN Phase I has completed fieldwork with data and methodology quality checks in a large number of centres in both high-income and low- or middle-income countries including representation from all inhabited continents. This broad geographical coverage is expected to expand as a number of centres have commenced fieldwork but not yet submitted completed data. However, four countries (India, Kosovo, Mexico and Spain) account for two-thirds of the datasets received by 31 May 2020 which may limit the international generalisability of the findings.

Overlap between ISAAC and GAN is less extensive than anticipated, but 21 diverse centres will provide local time-trends in disease prevalence. These within-centre trends can be used, with caution, to inform projections of trends in prevalence among the remaining centres in ISAAC Phase III, which offer a much more widespread international representation than has been achieved so far in GAN.

Careful checks of the methodology used (centre report and data checks), as with ISAAC, ensured clarity on how the study was actually done and any variations encountered. The high levels of responses achieved in ISAAC have generally been maintained in GAN, suggesting that estimates of prevalence and severity of asthma will be representative of the populations surveyed. Sample sizes in most centres achieved the recommended target of 3000 children per age group, leading to precise estimates of disease prevalence, but in a few centres the numbers of respondents are substantially lower (Table 2).

The response rate in both age groups in Guatemala was unusually low (Table 3) and we explored the possible reasons for this. In both age groups, questionnaires were sent home for completion by the parents, whereas in other centres, the adolescents self-completed the questionnaires in class. This probably explains the exceptionally low response rate among 13–14-year-olds in Guatemala.

Extension of ISAAC methodology to include questions about parental symptoms was an attempt to fill gaps in knowledge about the prevalence, severity, diagnosis and management of asthma and related risk factors among young and middle-aged adults. Parents of schoolchildren are not a random or representative sample of the adult population, but the high response rates achieved in many of the study centres suggest that useful results could be obtained in this manner. The total number of adult respondents in GAN (177,622) is comparable with two previous international studies of young and middle-aged adults, discussed below.

The ECRHS, (1991–1993) recruited 137,619 participants aged 20–44 years in 48 centres in 22 countries (including 5 non-European countries: Algeria, Australia, India, New Zealand, USA) [17]. The GAN adult questionnaire incorporates core ECRHS items, but the geographical overlap with ECRHS countries is limited. The World Health Survey (WHS, 2002–2003) interviewed 178,215 adults aged 18–45 years from 70 countries and included a few questions about asthma and related symptoms among a general health questionnaire [6]. Although there is better geographical overlap with GAN, at least at the country level, the WHS questionnaire lacks detail which limits the scope for historical comparisons with GAN data on asthma severity.

Among adolescents and children, ISAAC offered a global perspective on time trends in asthma prevalence from the mid-1990s to the early 2000s [5,18] but very few ISAAC centres have repeated their local surveys subsequently, prior to GAN. In Brazil, adolescents in Curitiba, Recife and São Paulo were studied in ISAAC Phases I (1994) and III (2003) and again in 2012 [19] and in South Santiago, Chile, ISAAC Phases I and III were completed, and a further survey of asthma in adolescents completed in 2015 [20]. Three GAN Phase I studies with previous ISAAC data have been published: in Bangkok, Thailand, [21] and four Mexican centres [22,23]. Time trends in these centres have been summarised elsewhere [8].

With the closure of this first round of data in GAN Phase I, these temporal and geographical comparisons can now be extended to a wider and more diverse range of study centres. These results will form the basis of analyses for journal publications in the near future. However, GAN centres that were unable to meet the criteria for this first data compilation can still contribute results to future analyses and publications. The GAN Phase I Study Group is listed at the Appendix A.

In summary, GAN Phase I offers, for the first time in nearly two decades, new standardised worldwide data on prevalence and severity of asthma in adolescents, children and adults. This will enable comparisons to be made over time, and contribute a new picture of the global burden of asthma, rhinoconjunctivitis and eczema. Not only will risk factors be examined, but also time trends in these, and global variation, shedding light on causation. The methodology which ISAAC started has a proven track record of over nearly 30 years, and now extends to adults (parents) as well as adolescents and children. The high response rates achieved in a range of settings are testimony to the feasibility of the approach and give confidence in the estimates obtained.

Author Contributions: Study design—P.E., E.E., M.I.A., L.G.-M., N.P., D.S., GAN Steering Group. Conduct—P.E., all study centres. Analysis—C.R., V.P.-F., E.M., E.E. Writing lead—D.S. Review of manuscript—all named authors. All authors have read and agreed to the published version of the manuscript.

Funding: This research received no external funding.

Acknowledgments: The GAN Global Centre in Auckland was funded by The University of Auckland, The International Union Against Tuberculosis and Lung Disease and Boehringer Ingelheim NZ. The London Data Centre was supported by a PhD studentship [to C.R.] from the UK Medical Research Council (grant number MR/N013638/1) and funding from the European Research Council under the European Union's Seventh Framework Programme (FP7/2007–2013, ERC grant agreement number 668954). The Murcia Data Centre was supported by the University of Murcia and by Instituto de Salud Carlos III, fund PI17/0170. Individual centres involved in GAN Phase I data collection were funded by the following organisations: Brazil, Uruguaiana, Funded by Marilyn Urrutia Pereira; Cameroon, Yaounde, funded by Elvis Ndikum (95%) and from family, friends (5%); Costa Rica, Guatemala, Honduras and Nicaragua partially funded by an unrestricted grant from Astra Zenica for logistic purposes. India; Kottayam, New Delhi, Chandigarh, Bikaner, Jaipur, Lucknow, Kolkata, Pune, Mysuru, GAN Phase I was undertaken by Asthma Bhawan in India which was supported by Cipla Foundation; Iran: Karaj, funded by the Alborz University of Medical Sciences; Kosovo, Gjakova, Municipality of Gjakova and the Directorate for Health and Education; Mexico, Puerto Vallarta Centro Universitario de la Costa, Universidad de Guadalajara; New Zealand, Auckland Asthma Charitable Trust; Nigeria, Ibadan, funded by National Institute for Health Research (NIHR) (IMPALA grant Ref 16/136/35) using UK aid from the UK Government to support Global Health Research; Poland, Katowice funded by the Medical University of Silesia; South Africa, Cape Town, SA Medical Research Council, Allergy Society of South Africa; Spain, Salamanca, Gerencia Regional de Salud. Junta de Castilla y León. España, Sociedad Española de Inmunología Clínica, Alergología y Asma Pediátrica. (SEICAP); Sri Lanka; Anuradhapura, Peradeniya, University of Peradeniya, Peradeniya, Sri Lanka; Syria; Damascus, Lattakia, Damascus: Syrian Private University, Lattakia: Lattakia Medical Syndicate.

Conflicts of Interest: The authors declare no conflict of interest.

Appendix A

GAN Phase I Study Group

Global Asthma Network Steering Group: I Asher, University of Auckland, Auckland, New Zealand; N Billo, Joensuu, Finland; K Bissell, School of Population Health, University of Auckland, Auckland, New Zealand; Chiang C-Y, Division of Pulmonary Medicine, Department of Internal Medicine, Wan Fang Hospital, Taipei Medical University, Taipei, Taiwan; A El Sony, The Epidemiological Laboratory for Public Health and Research, Khartoum, Sudan; P Ellwood, University of Auckland, Auckland, New Zealand; L García-Marcos, Virgen de la Arrixaca University Children's Hospital, Murcia, Spain; J Mallol, University of Santiago de Chile (USACH), Santiago, Chile; G Marks, University of New South Wales, Sydney, Australia; K Mortimer, Liverpool School of Tropical Medicine and Aintree University Hospital NHS Foundation Trust, Liverpool, United Kingdom; N Pearce, London School of Hygiene and Tropical Medicine, London, United Kingdom; D Strachan, St George's, University of London, London, United Kingdom.

Global Asthma Network International Data Centres: Auckland: P Ellwood, E Ellwood, I Asher, University of Auckland, Auckland, New Zealand; **Murcia:** V Pérez-Fernández, E Morales, University of Murcia, Murcia, Spain; L García-Marcos, Pediatric Allergy and Pulmonology Units, 'Virgen de la Arrixaca' University Children's Hospital, University of Murcia, ARADyAL network and Biomedical

Research Institute of Murcia (IMIB-Arrixaca), Murcia, Spain; **London:** C Rutter, R Silverwood, S Robertson, Neil Pearce, London School of Hygiene & Tropical Medicine, London, United Kingdom; D Strachan, St George's, University of London, London, United Kingdom.

Global Asthma Network Principal Investigators: Brazil: M Urrutia-Pereira, Federal University of Pampa, UNIPAMPA (Uruguaiana); Cameroon: AE Ndikum, The University of Yaounde 1 (Yaounde); Costa Rica: ME Soto-Quirós, University of Costa Rica (Costa Rica); Greece: K Douros, National and Kapodistrian University of Athens (Athens); Guatemala: L Pérez-Martini, Asociación Guatemalteca de Neumología y Cirugía de Tórax (Guatemala City); Honduras: SM Sosa Ferrari, Instituto Nacional Cardiopulmonar (Tegucigalpa); India: M Sabir, Maharaja Agrasen Medical College Agroha (Bikaner); M Singh, Postgraduate Institute of Medical Education and Research (Chandigarh); V Singh*, Asthma Bhawan (Jaipur); AG Ghoshal, National Allergy Asthma Bronchitis Institute (Kolkata (19)); TU Sukumaran, PIMS Thiruvalla (Kottayam); S Awasthi, King George's Medical University (Lucknow); PA Mahesh, JSS University (Mysuru); SK Kabra, All India Institute of Medical Sciences (New Delhi); S Salvi, Chest Research Foundation (Pune); Iran: M Tavakol, Alborz University of Medical Sciences (Karaj); N Behniafard, Shahid Sadoughi University of Medical Sciences (Yazd); Kosovo: I Bucaliu-Ismajli, The principal center of family care (Ferizaj); L Pajaziti, (Gjakova); V Gashi, American Hospital in Kosovo (Gjilan); LN Ahmetaj*, University Hospital of Prishtina (Prishtina); V Zhjeqi, University of Prishtina (Prizren); Mexico: MG Sanchez Coronel, COMPEDIA (Colegio Mexicano de Pediatras (Aguascalientes); HL Moreno Gardea, Hospital Angeles Chihuahua (Chihuahua); G Ochoa-Lopez, Department of Pediatric Allergology (Ciudad Juárez); R García-Almaráz, Hospital Infantil de Tamaulipas (Ciudad Victoria); JA Sacre Hazouri, Instituto Privado de Alergia, (Córdoba); DD Hernández-Colín, Hospital Civil De Guadalajara Juan I Menchaca (Guadalajara); N Rodriguez-Perez, Instituto de Ciencias y Estudios Superiores de Tamaulipas (Matamoros); JV Mérida-Palacio, Centro de Investigacion de Enfermedades Alergicas y Respiratorias (Mexicali); BE Del Río Navarro*, Service of Allergy and Clinical immunology, Hospital Infantil de México (Mexico City North); LO Hernández-Mondragón, CRIT de Michoacán (Michoacán); Md Juan Pineda, Universidad de Guadalajara (Puerto Vallarta); Bd Ramos García, Instituto Mexicano del Seguro Social (San Luis Potosí); AJ Escalante-Dominguez, Hospital General Tijuana [Isesalud] (Tijuana); EM Navarrete-Rodriguez, Hospital Infantil de Mexico Federico Gomez (Toluca Urban); FJ Linares-Zapién, Centro De Enfermedades Alergicas Y Asma de Toluca (Toluca Rural); J Santos Lozano, Medica san Angel (Xalapa); New Zealand: I Asher, University of Auckland (Auckland); Nicaragua: JF Sánchez, Hospital Infantil Manuel de Jesús Rivera (Managua); Nigeria: AG Falade, University of Ibadan and University College Hospital (Ibadan); Poland: G Brożek, Medical University of Silesia (Katowice); South Africa: HJ Zar, SA MRC Unit on Child & Adolescent Health (Cape Town); Spain: A Bercedo Sanz, Cantabrian Health Service (Cantabria); L García-Marcos*, Pediatric Allergy and Pulmonology Units, 'Virgen de la Arrixaca' University Children's Hospital, University of Murcia, ARADyAL network and Biomedical Research Institute of Murcia (IMIB-Arrixaca), Murcia, Spain (Cartagena); A López-Silvarrey Varela, Fundacion Maria Jose Jove (La Coruña); J Pellegrini Belinchon, Universidad de Salamanca (Salamanca); Sri Lanka: JC Ranasinghe, Teaching Hospital Peradeniya (Anuradhapura); ST Kudagammana, University of Peradeniya (Peradeniya); Syrian Arab Republic: G Alkhayer, Damascus Private University (Damascus); G Dib, Lattakia University (Lattakia 13–14); Y Mohammad*, National Center for research and training for chronic respiratory disease and co_morbidities (Lattakia 6–7); Taiwan: J-L Huang, Chang Gung University (Taipei); Thailand: P Vichyanond*, Mahidol University (Bangkok).

* National Coordinators

Global Asthma Network Adult Age Group Principal Investigators not named above:

Cameroon: GA Ajeagah, The University of Yaounde 1 (Yaounde); Costa Rica: M Soto-Martinez, University of Costa Rica (Costa Rica); Greece: K Priftis, National and Kapodistrian University of Athens (Athens); Guatemala: M Cohen-Todd, Asociacion Guatemalteca De Neumologia Y Cirugia De Torax (Guatemala City); Honduras: J Sanchez, Instituto Nacional Cardiopulmonar (Tegucigalpa); India: SK Kochar, Sardar Patel Medical College (Bikaner); N Singh, Asthma Bhawan (Jaipur); N Sit, National

Allergy Asthma Bronchitis Institute (Kolkata (19)); S Sinha, All India Institute of Medical Sciences (New Delhi); M Barne, Chest Research Foundation (Pune); Kosovo: B Ajeti, The Principal center of Family Care (Ferizaj); LH Lleshi, (Gjakova); V Lokaj-Berisha, University of Prishtina (Prizren); Mexico: Md Ambriz-Moreno, (Matamoros); OJ Saucedo-Ramirez, Hospital Angeles Pedregal (Mexico City North); CA Jiménez González, Universidad Autonoma of San Luis Potosí (San Luis Potosí); Taiwan: K-W Yeh, (Taipei); Thailand: S Chinratanapisit, Bhumibol Adulyadej Hospital (Bangkok).

Global Asthma Network National Co-ordinators not named above: Brasil: D Solé, Escola Paulista de Medicina, Federal University of São Paulo, São Paulo.

ISAAC Phase III Principal Investigators: Costa Rica: ME Soto-Quirós*, University of Costa Rica (Costa Rica); India: M Sabir, Maharaja Agrasen Medical College Agroha (Bikaner); L Kumar†, Department of Pediatrics (Chandigarh); V Singh, Asthma Bhawan (Jaipur); T Sukumaran, PIMS Thiruvalla (Kottayam); S Awasthi, King George's Medical University (Lucknow); SK Sharma, All India Institute of Medical Sciences (New Delhi (7)); NM Hanumante, Ruby Hall Clinic (Pune); Mexico: R García-Almaráz, Hospital Infantil de Tamaulipas (Ciudad Victoria); JV Merida-Palacio, Centro de Investigacion de Enfermedades Alergicas y Respiratorias (Mexicali Valley); BE Del-Río-Navarro, Service of Allergy and Clinical immunology, Hospital Infantil de México (Ciudad de México (1)); FJ Linares-Zapién, Centro De Enfermedades Alergicas Y Asma de Toluca (Toluca); New Zealand: MI Asher*, University of Auckland (Auckland); Nicaragua: JF Sánchez*, Hospital Infantil Manuel de Jesús Rivera (Managua); Nigeria: BO Onadeko, (Ibadan); South Africa: HJ Zar*, University of Cape Town (Cape Town); Spain: L García-Marcos*, Pediatric Allergy and Pulmonology Units, 'Virgen de la Arrixaca' University Children's Hospital, University of Murcia, ARADyAL network and Biomedical Research Institute of Murcia (IMIB-Arrixaca), Murcia, Spain (Cartagena); A López-Silvarrey Varela, Fundacion Maria Jose Jove (A Coruña); Syria: Y Mohammad, National Center for Research and Training in Chronic Respiratory Diseases—Tishreen University (Lattakia); Taiwan: J-L Huang*, Chang Gung University (Taipei); Thailand: P Vichyanond*, Mahidol University (Bangkok).

* National Coordinators
† Deceased

ISAAC Phase III National Co-ordinators not named above: Mexico: M Baeza-Bacab, University Autónoma de Yucatán, Yucatán; Syrian Arab Republic: S Mohammad, Tishreen University, Lattakia.

ISAAC Phase I Principal Investigators: Costa Rica: ME Soto-Quirós*, University of Costa Rica (Costa Rica); Greece: CH Gratziou*, National Kapodistrian University of Athens (Athens); India: L Kumar, Department of Pediatrics (Chandigarh); T Sukumaran, PIMS Thiruvalla (Kottayam); K Chopra, Maulana Azad Medical College (New Delhi (7)); NM Hanumante, Ruby Hall Clinic (Pune); New Zealand: MI Asher*, University of Auckland (Auckland); Nigeria: BO Onadeko, (Ibadan); Spain: L García-Marcos*, Pediatric Allergy and Pulmonology Units, 'Virgen de la Arrixaca' University Children's Hospital, University of Murcia, ARADyAL network and Biomedical Research Institute of Murcia (IMIB-Arrixaca), Murcia, Spain (Cartagena); Taiwan: K-H Hsieh†, Chang Gung Children's Hospital (Taipei); Thailand: P Vichyanond*, Mahidol University (Bangkok); South Africa: R Erlich, University of Cape Town (Cape Town);

* National Coordinators
† Deceased

ISAAC Phase I National Co-ordinators not named above: India: J Shah, Jaslok Hospital & Research Centre, Mumbai.

References

1. Global Asthma Network. Available online: http://www.globalasthmanetwork.org (accessed on 17 November 2020).

2. Ellwood, P.; Asher, M.I.; Billo, N.E.; Bissell, K.; Chiang, C.Y.; Ellwood, E.M.; El-Sony, A.; García-Marcos, L.; Mallol, J.; Marks, G.B.; et al. The Global Asthma Network rationale and methods for Phase I global surveillance: Prevalence, severity, management and risk factors. *Eur. Respir. J.* **2017**, *49*, 1601635. [CrossRef]
3. *The Global Asthma Report 2011*; The International Union Against Tuberculosis and Lung Disease: Paris, France, 2011; ISBN 978-2-914365-83-3.
4. Lai, C.K.W.; Beasley, R.; Crane, J.; Foliaki, S.; Shah, J.; Weiland, S. ISAAC Phase Three Study Group. Global variation in the prevalence and severity of asthma symptoms: Phase Three of the International Study of Asthma and Allergies in Childhood (ISAAC). *Thorax* **2009**, *64*, 476–483. [CrossRef] [PubMed]
5. Pearce, N.; Aït-Khaled, N.; Beasley, R.; Mallol, J.; Keil, U.; Mitchell, E.; Robertson, C.; ISAAC Phase Three Study Group. Worldwide trends in the prevalence of asthma symptoms: Phase III of the International Study of Asthma and Allergies in Childhood (ISAAC). *Thorax* **2007**, *62*, 758–766. [CrossRef] [PubMed]
6. Sembajwe, G.; Cifuentes, M.; Tak, S.W.; Kriebel, D.; Gore, R.; Punnett, L. National income, self-reported wheezing and asthma diagnosis from the World Health Survey. *Eur. Respir. J.* **2010**, *35*, 279–286. [CrossRef] [PubMed]
7. *The Global Asthma Report 2018*; Global Asthma Network: Auckland, New Zealand, 2018; ISBN 978-0-473-46523-0/978-0-473-46524-7.
8. Asher, I.; Garcia-Marcos, L.; Pearce, N.; Strachan, D. Trends in worldwide asthma prevalence. *Eur. Respir. J.* **2020**, in press. [CrossRef] [PubMed]
9. WHO Model Lists of Essential Medicines. Available online: https://www.who.int/medicines/publications/essentialmedicines/en/ (accessed on 17 November 2020).
10. *The Global Asthma Report 2014*; Global Asthma Network: Auckland, New Zealand, 2014; pp. 44–57. ISBN 978-0-473-29125-9/978-0-473-29126-6.
11. Asher, I.; Haahtela, T.; Selroos, O.; Ellwood, P.; Ellwood, E.; The Global Asthma Study Network Group. Global Asthma Network survey suggests more national asthma strategies could reduce burden of asthma. *Allergol. Immunopathol.* **2017**, *45*, 105–114. [CrossRef] [PubMed]
12. Bissell, K.; Ellwood, P.; Ellwood, E.; Chiang, C.Y.; Marks, G.B.; El Sony, A.; Asher, I.; Billo, N.; Perrin, C.; The Global Asthma Network Study Group. Essential medicines at the national level: The Global Asthma Network's essential asthma medicines survey 2014. *Int. J. Environ. Res. Public Health* **2019**, *16*, 605. [CrossRef] [PubMed]
13. Ellwood, P.; Ellwood, E.; Asher, I. Asthma management guidelines and strategies—Who has them? *Am. J. Respir. Crit. Care Med.* **2014**, *189*, A104.
14. Ellwood, P.; Asher, M.I.; Ellwood, E.; Global Asthma Network Steering Group. *Manual for Global Surveillance: Prevalence, Severity and Risk Factors*; Global Asthma Network Data Centre: Auckland, New Zealand, 2015; ISBN 978-0-473-31442-2.
15. Ellwood, P.; Williams, H.; Ait-Khaled, N.; Bjorksten, B.; Robertson, C.; Group IPIS. Translation of questions: The International Study of Asthma and Allergies in Childhood (ISAAC) experience. *Int. J. Tuberc. Lung Dis.* **2009**, *13*, 1174–1182. [PubMed]
16. Crane, J.; Mallol, J.; Beasley, R.; Stewart, A.; Asher, M.I. Agreement between written and video questions for comparing asthma symptoms in ISAAC. *Eur. Respir. J.* **2003**, *21*, 455–461. [CrossRef] [PubMed]
17. Burney, P.G.J.; Luczynska, C.; Chinn, S.; Jarvis, D. The European Community Respiratory Health Survey. *Eur. Respir. J.* **1994**, *7*, 954–960. [CrossRef] [PubMed]
18. Asher, M.I.; Montefort, S.; Björkstén, B.; Lai, C.K.; Strachan, D.P.; Weiland, S.K.; Williams, H.; the ISAAC Phase Three Study Group. Worldwide time trends in the prevalence of symptoms of asthma, allergic rhinoconjunctivitis, and eczema in childhood: ISAAC Phases One and Three repeat multicountry cross-sectional surveys. *Lancet* **2006**, *368*, 733–743. [CrossRef]
19. Sole, D.; Rosario Filho, N.; Sarinho, E.C.; Silva, A.R.; Britto, M.; Riedi, C.; Cardozo, C.; Camelo-Nunes, I.C.; De Andrade, D.; Mallol, J. Prevalence of asthma and related symptoms in adolescents: Findings from 3 surveys. *J. Investig. Allergol. Clin. Immunol.* **2015**, *25*, 73–74. [PubMed]
20. Mallol, J.; Aguirre, V.; Mallol-Simmonds, M.; Matamala-Bezmalinovic, A.; Calderon-Rodriguez, L.; Osses-Vergara, F. Changes in the prevalence of asthma and related risk factors in adolescents: Three surveys between 1994 and 2015. *Allergol. Immunopathol.* **2019**, *47*, 313–321. [CrossRef] [PubMed]

21. Chinratanapisit, S.; Suratannon, N.; Pacharn, P.; Sritipsukho, P.; Vichyanond, P. Prevalence and severity of asthma, rhinoconjunctivitis and eczema in children from the Bangkok area: The Global Asthma Network (GAN) Phase, I. *Asian Pac. J. Allergy Immunol.* **2019**, *37*, 226–231. [PubMed]
22. Del-Rio-Navarro, B.E.; Navarrete Rodríguez, E.M.; Berber, A.; Reyes-Noriega, N.; García-Marcos Álvarez, L.; Grupo GAN México; Grupo ISAAC México. The burden of asthma in an inner-city area: A historical review 10 years after ISAAC. *World Allergy Org. J.* **2020**, *13*, 100092. [CrossRef] [PubMed]
23. Del-Rio-Navarro, B.E.; Berber, A.; Noriega, N.R.; Navarrete Rodríguez, E.M.; García Almaráz, R.; Mérida Palacio, J.V.; Ellwood, P.; García-Marcos, L. What are the time trends in the prevalence of asthma symptoms in Mexico? *Allergol. Immunopathol.* **2020**, in press.

Publisher's Note: MDPI stays neutral with regard to jurisdictional claims in published maps and institutional affiliations.

© 2020 by the authors. Licensee MDPI, Basel, Switzerland. This article is an open access article distributed under the terms and conditions of the Creative Commons Attribution (CC BY) license (http://creativecommons.org/licenses/by/4.0/).

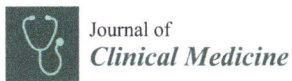

Article

Longitudinal Asthma Patterns in Italian Adult General Population Samples: Host and Environmental Risk Factors

Sara Maio [1,*], Sandra Baldacci [1], Marzia Simoni [1], Anna Angino [1], Stefania La Grutta [2], Vito Muggeo [3], Salvatore Fasola [2], Giovanni Viegi [1,2] and on behalf of the AGAVE Pisa Group [†]

1. Pulmonary Environmental Epidemiology Unit, CNR Institute of Clinical Physiology (IFC), 56126 Pisa, Italy; baldas@ifc.cnr.it (S.B.); marzia_simoni@libero.it (M.S.); anginoa@ifc.cnr.it (A.A.); giovanni.viegi@irib.cnr.it (G.V.)
2. CNR Institute for Biomedical Research and Innovation (IRIB), 90146 Palermo, Italy; stefania.lagrutta@irib.cnr.it (S.L.G.); salvatore.fasola@irib.cnr.it (S.F.)
3. Department of Economics, Business and Statistics, University of Palermo, 90128 Palermo, Italy; vito.muggeo@unipa.it
* Correspondence: saramaio@ifc.cnr.it
† AGAVE Pisa Group: CNR Institute of Clinical Physiology, Pisa: A. Angino; S. Baldacci; M. Bresciani; L. Carrozzi; S. Cerrai; S. Maio; F. Martini; A.P. Pala; F. Pistelli; G. Sarno; P. Silvi; M. Simoni; G. Viegi.

Received: 28 September 2020; Accepted: 9 November 2020; Published: 11 November 2020

Abstract: Background: Asthma patterns are not well established in epidemiological studies. Aim: To assess asthma patterns and risk factors in an adult general population sample. Methods: In total, 452 individuals reporting asthma symptoms/diagnosis in previous surveys participated in the AGAVE survey (2011–2014). Latent transition analysis (LTA) was performed to detect baseline and 12-month follow-up asthma phenotypes and longitudinal patterns. Risk factors associated with longitudinal patterns were assessed through multinomial logistic regression. Results: LTA detected four longitudinal patterns: persistent asthma diagnosis with symptoms, 27.2%; persistent asthma diagnosis without symptoms, 4.6%; persistent asthma symptoms without diagnosis, 44.0%; and ex-asthma, 24.1%. The longitudinal patterns were differently associated with asthma comorbidities. Persistent asthma diagnosis with symptoms showed associations with passive smoke (OR 2.64, 95% CI 1.10–6.33) and traffic exposure (OR 1.86, 95% CI 1.02–3.38), while persistent asthma symptoms (without diagnosis) with passive smoke (OR 3.28, 95% CI 1.41–7.66) and active smoke (OR 6.24, 95% CI 2.68–14.51). Conclusions: LTA identified three cross-sectional phenotypes and their four longitudinal patterns in a real-life setting. The results highlight the necessity of a careful monitoring of exposure to active/passive smoke and vehicular traffic, possible determinants of occurrence of asthma symptoms (with or without diagnosis). Such information could help affected patients and physicians in prevention and management strategies.

Keywords: asthma; epidemiology; cohort; latent transition analysis; comorbidities; smoke; vehicular traffic

1. Introduction

Asthma prevalence has reached epidemic proportions (1–18%) [1] due to host and environmental risk factors [2,3].

According to the Global Burden of Disease Study, in 2017, total deaths from asthma were 495,000 globally [4]; all-age prevalent cases of asthma were 273 million and all-age incident cases were 43 million (about 50% and 70% of all the chronic respiratory diseases, respectively) [5].

Asthma may begin at any age (mainly in children). It may clinically persist, conclusively remit, or present combination of remissions and relapses over time [6–8]; as a result, its course is difficult to characterize and its prognosis difficult to predict [7]. In adults, asthma that has persisted from childhood is potentially difficult to treat and it is a distinct clinical phenotype; however, characteristics of these patients are not well documented [9]. A thorough characterization of adult patients with persistent asthma and their risk factors may help clinicians in establishing treatment plans and applying preventive interventions [9,10]. Indeed, from a clinical perspective, it is essential to elucidate the asthma natural history and long-term outcomes; studies on asthmatic cohorts can help [6].

Moreover, although asthma control can be achieved in the majority of patients participating in controlled trials, available data show that this is not the case in real-life [11]; thus, it becomes important to deepen the knowledge in this setting.

Disentangling respiratory diseases phenotypes is a current research challenge [8,12,13], and "unsupervised" or "data-driven" approaches have been proposed. These approaches may allow defining objective, novel, or previously unrecognized phenotypes, by using clustering algorithms accounting for multiple disease features [14,15]. In particular, latent transition analysis (LTA) is a statistical method that can incorporate the longitudinal patterns of several disease manifestations into a comprehensive statistical model, which simultaneously defines phenotypes and their changes over time [12,14]. When disease prevalence changes over time, transition probabilities can help explain the dynamics of such change [14]. However, most studies on asthma phenotyping using data-driven methods involve patients with moderate to severe asthma and/or clinical settings, which limits the possibility of generalizing the findings to the general population [15].

In this framework, data of the AGAVE survey ("Severe Asthma: epidemiological and clinical cohorts follow up by registry and questionnaires; therapeutic appropriateness and outcome assessment, according to GINA guidelines") were analyzed.

The AGAVE survey, funded by the Italian Medicines Agency (AIFA), was carried out during 2011–2014 to assess asthma modifiable risk factors and the effectiveness of therapeutic strategies, in epidemiological and clinical samples, through the implementation of an online registry [16].

This manuscript focuses on the AGAVE epidemiological sample, with the aim of assessing cross-sectional asthma phenotypes, their longitudinal patterns, and the associated risk factors.

2. Materials and Methods

2.1. Study Population

A randomized general population sample, living in the rural Po Delta area, North Italy, was involved in two subsequent cross-sectional surveys: first survey (1980–1982), 3284 subjects, and second survey (1988–1991), 2841 subjects. In total, 2136 subjects participated in both surveys [17].

The same protocol and selection method were used to enroll a random general population sample living in the urban and suburban area of Pisa, Central Italy, involved in three subsequent cross-sectional surveys: first survey (1985–1988), 3865 subjects; second survey (1991–1993), 2841 subjects; and third survey (2009–2011), 1620 subjects [18]. Overall, 2257 subjects participated in both the first and the second surveys, 1107 subjects in both the second and the third surveys, and 849 in all three Pisa surveys [18].

In the AGAVE survey (2011–2014), all subjects reporting asthma diagnosis or asthma symptoms (asthma attacks or wheezing) in any of the previous epidemiological surveys were invited: 68% agreed to participate ($n = 668$). In total, 454 subjects were investigated at both AGAVE baseline and follow-up. In this manuscript, only subjects having a baseline age of ≥16 years were taken into account ($n = 452$) (Figure 1).

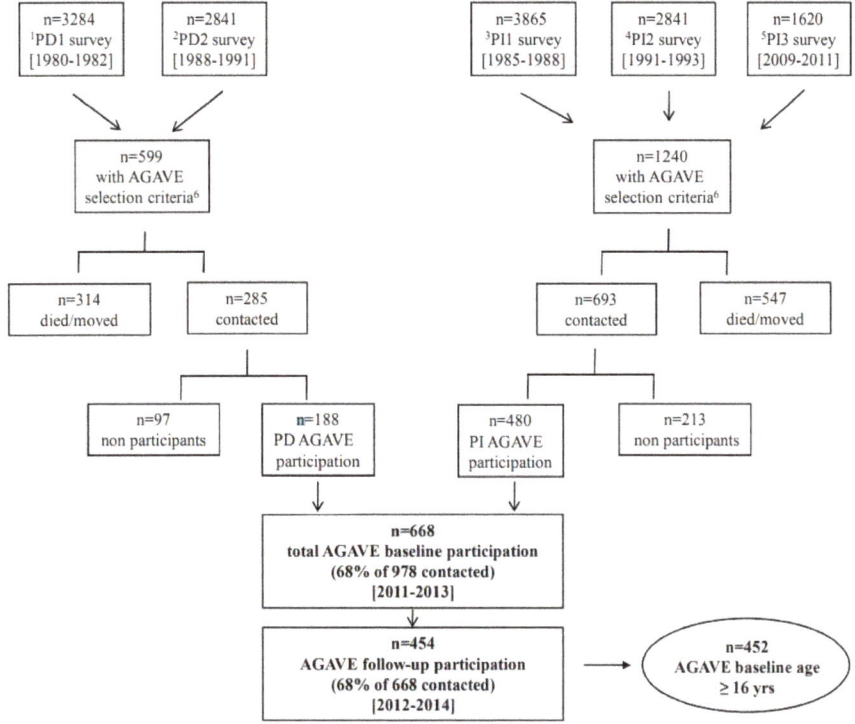

Figure 1. Flow-chart of subjects participation. [1]PD1, Po Delta first survey; [2]PD2, Po Delta second survey; [3]PI1, Pisa first survey; [4]PI2, Pisa second survey; [5]PI3, Pisa third survey; [6]AGAVE selection criteria: subjects reporting asthma diagnosis or asthma symptoms (asthma attacks or wheezing) in at least one of the previous epidemiological surveys.

2.2. Data Collection Tool

Each subject underwent a telephone interview lasting about 20 min, based on a questionnaire covering the main items of the GINA guidelines [1], which include asthma symptoms, treatment, exacerbation, symptom control, comorbidity, and exposure to risk factors. The questions were derived from different validated questionnaires such as the European Community Respiratory Health Survey (ECRHS) questionnaire [19] and those used by our research group in other surveys about respiratory health [20–22]. The latter were derived from the National Heart Lung and Blood Institute (NHLBI, Bethesda, MD, USA) questionnaire. The AGAVE questionnaire was reviewed and approved by an interdisciplinary internal board, comprised of pulmonologists, allergists, and epidemiologists.

The AGAVE epidemiological questionnaire investigates: asthma clinical history, asthma diagnosis, and use of health services due to asthma throughout life; asthma symptoms, comorbidities, exacerbations, and use of health services due to asthma in the last 12-months; asthma symptoms, asthma control, and asthma treatment in the last month; and current exposure to risk factors.

The same questionnaire was used in the first and second interviews allowing to collect the answers to repeated questions in a longitudinal fashion.

An extract of the AGAVE epidemiological questionnaire, reporting the questions used to define the variables in this manuscript, is available in the Supplementary Materials.

The AGAVE study protocol, patient information sheet, and consent form were approved by the Ethics Committee of the Pisa University Hospital (Prot. No. 17658, 21 March 2011).

2.3. Statistical Analyses

Statistical analyses were carried out using the Statistical Package for the Social Sciences (SPSS version 26.0) and the R software (version 3.5.1). Comparisons among groups were performed by Chi-square test for categorical variables and analysis of variance for continuous variables. The significance level was set at 0.05.

Post-hoc analyses were run to assess the sources of statistically significant results, using adjusted standardized residuals for contingency tables larger than the 2 × 2.

LTA was performed using the R package CAT_LVM (Version 0.9.0 alpha, available at https://msu.edu/~chunghw/downloads.html). The main advantage of LTA, over other clustering techniques, is its ability to incorporate into a comprehensive statistical model information about possible changes in the disease characteristics over time, in a longitudinal fashion. Indeed, differently from cross-sectional analytical approaches such as latent class analysis [23], LTA requires temporal variability in all the variables and is much more indicated for characterizing transitions over time [24]. LTA detects unobservable (latent) subgroups ("classes" or "phenotypes") of subjects based on the values of multiple observed (or "manifest") variables. The latent classes are exhaustive and mutually exclusive, and they are not assumed to be stable over time. Indeed, LTA also estimates the probabilities of transitions from one latent class to another between different time points [25].

The characterization of asthma (cross-sectional) phenotypes was based on the presence/absence of asthma outcomes, measured at AGAVE baseline and 12-month follow-up (manifest variables), defined as follows: previous physician diagnosed asthma, if the subject answered "YES, but I no longer have it" to the question "Has your doctor ever told you that you have bronchial asthma?"; current physician diagnosed asthma, if the subject answered "YES, I still have it" to the question "Has your doctor ever told you that you have bronchial asthma?"; current asthma attacks if the subject answered "YES" to the question "During the past 12 months, have you had attacks of shortness of breath with wheezing or whistling, apart from common colds?"; and current wheeze if the subject answered "YES" to the question "During the past 12 months, have you had wheezing or whistling, apart from common colds?".

The model with the lowest Bayesian Information Criterion (BIC), i.e., associated with the best balance of model fit and parsimony, was selected; at each time point, the subjects were assigned to the phenotype associated with the maximum posterior probability of latent class membership [25]. Thus, the longitudinal patterns were defined based on the observed phenotype transitions.

Host and environmental risk factors associated with the longitudinal asthma patterns were assessed through multinomial logistic regression. Only significant variables were retained in the regression analysis to obtain a parsimonious model and improve the statistical power.

Sensitivity analyses were performed comparing AGAVE asthma phenotypes to those of the previous epidemiological surveys from which AGAVE subjects were selected.

3. Results

3.1. Baseline Subject Characteristics

In total, 452 subjects aged ≥16 years, and participating in both the interviews, were included in the analyses (Table 1). As regards the time frame, the target was 12 months between the first and second questionnaires within a study period of 24 months. The actual result was a mean interval of 15 ± 4 months between the two interviews.

The mean age was 56.7 years; most subjects were females (52.7%), with a middle-low educational level. Fifty-one percent of subjects were overweight–obese (Table 1).

About 75% of the subjects reported skin prick test positivity and about 40% family history of asthma (Table 2).

Table 1. Baseline descriptive characteristics of the investigated subjects ($n = 452$).

Gender (%):	
Males	47.3
Females	52.7
Age (mean ± SD [1]) (years)	56.7 ± 15.5
Age range (min-max)	17–91
BMI [2] (kg/m^2) groups [3] (%):	
obese (BMI ≥ 30 kg/m^2)	15.7
overweight (BMI 25.0–29.9 kg/m^2)	35.3
normal weight (BMI 18.5–24.9 kg/m^2)	46.6
underweight (BMI < 18.5 kg/m^2)	2.4
Educational level (%):	
elementary/junior high school	45.2
high school	35.9
university	18.9

[1] SD, standard deviation; [2] BMI, body mass index; [3] threshold values recommended by WHO.

Table 2. Baseline host and environmental risk factors of the investigated subjects ($n = 452$).

Host Risk Factors	
Reported SPT [1] positivity (%)	74.9
Family history of asthma (%)	40.7
Allergic rhinitis (%)	40.8
GERD [2] (%)	29.6
Sleep apnea (%)	14.7
Recurrent respiratory infections (%)	13.5
COPD [3] (%)	12.5
Nasal polyps (%)	3.4
Environmental Risk Factors	
Traffic exposure at home address (%)	58.4
Smoking habits (%):	
current smokers	19.4
ex-smokers	40.3
Pack-years in current smokers (mean ± SD [4]), n	23.6 ± 17.7
Pack-years in ex-smokers (mean ± SD [4]), n	27.2 ± 27.9
Secondhand smoke exposure (%)	17.4

[1] SPT, skin prick test (only subjects performing skin prick test $n = 211$); [2] GERD, Gastroesophageal reflux disease; [3] COPD, chronic obstructive pulmonary disease; [4] SD, standard deviation.

The most frequent asthma comorbidity was allergic rhinitis (40.8%), followed by gastroesophageal reflux disease (GERD) (29.6%), sleep apnea, recurrent respiratory infections, and chronic obstructive pulmonary disease (COPD) (about 13–14%); very few reported nasal polyps (Table 2).

Over 50% of subjects were exposed to vehicular traffic near home, 40.3% were ex-smokers, and 19.4% current smokers. Less than 20% of subjects were exposed to secondhand smoke (Table 2).

3.2. Asthma Phenotypes

Three cross-sectional phenotypes were detected by LTA and labeled as: "asthma diagnosis and current asthma symptoms" due to the very high probability of asthma symptoms (from 50.4% to 73.8%) and diagnosis (about 100%) in the model; "current asthma symptoms" due to the high probability of asthma symptoms (from 10% to 32%) and very low probability of asthma diagnosis (0–1.5%); and "previous asthma diagnosis" due to the low probability of symptoms (0–12%) and very high probability of previous asthma diagnosis (about 100%). The most frequent phenotype was "current asthma symptoms" at both baseline and follow-up (about 45%), followed by "asthma diagnosis and current asthma symptoms" at baseline and "previous asthma diagnosis" at follow-up (Table 3).

Table 3. Asthma symptoms/diagnosis frequency (%) within each cross-sectional phenotype.

	Baseline			Follow-Up		
	Asthma Diagnosis and Current Asthma Symptoms (28.5%)	Current Asthma Symptoms (45.6%)	Previous Asthma Diagnosis (25.9%)	Asthma Diagnosis and Current Asthma Symptoms (27.0%)	Current Asthma Symptoms (44.2%)	Previous Asthma Diagnosis (28.8%)
Current wheeze	64.8	30.2	12	73.8	32	9.2
Current asthma attacks	57.4	10.2	0	50.4	13.5	3.1
Current asthma diagnosis	85.3	0	0	86.1	1.5	0.8
Previous asthma diagnosis	14.7	0	100	11.5	0	99.2

The transition plot showed a high stability of phenotypes from baseline to follow-up, ranging from 86.8% for "asthma diagnosis and current asthma symptoms" to 96.6% for "current asthma symptoms". In addition, 93.2% of subjects showed a long-term asthma remission, reporting no more asthma symptoms or diagnosis with respect to the previous epidemiological studies: this indicates an elevated stability of "previous asthma diagnosis" cross-sectional phenotype (Figure 2).

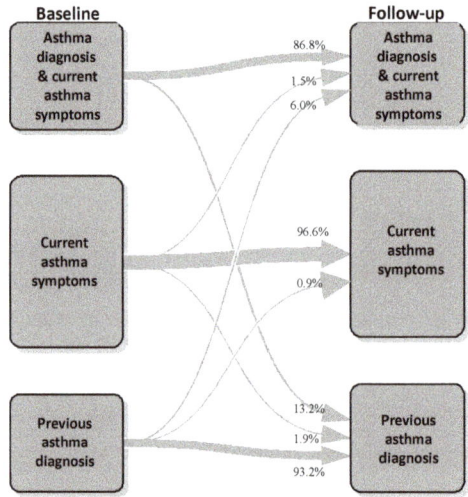

Figure 2. AGAVE phenotype transition plot.

Indeed, 13.2% of subjects showed an improvement of asthma status (from "asthma diagnosis and current asthma symptoms" to "previous asthma diagnosis") and 6% a worsening of asthma status in the last 12 months (from "previous asthma diagnosis" to "asthma diagnosis and current asthma symptoms"). At last, 1.5% of subjects reported a new asthma diagnosis in the last 12 months (from "current asthma symptoms" to "asthma diagnosis and current asthma symptoms") (Figure 2).

Based on the transition plot (Figure 2), the following longitudinal patterns were defined: "persistent asthma diagnosis with persistent/incident asthma symptoms", i.e., subjects with asthma diagnosis reporting asthma symptoms (wheeze or asthma attacks) at both baseline and follow-up or reporting new asthma symptoms at follow-up (27.2%); "persistent asthma diagnosis with remittent asthma symptoms", i.e., subjects with asthma diagnosis reporting asthma symptoms at baseline but not at follow-up (4.6%); "persistent asthma symptoms without asthma diagnosis", i.e., subjects reporting only asthma symptoms, without lifetime asthma diagnosis, at both baseline and follow-up (44.0%); and "ex-asthma", i.e., subjects reporting "previous asthma diagnosis" at both baseline and follow-up (24.1%) (Figure 3).

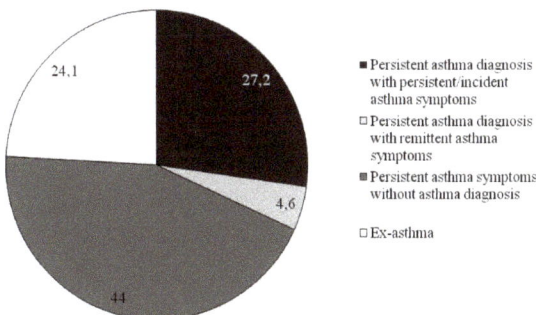

Figure 3. Longitudinal asthma patterns.

3.3. Subject Characteristics by Asthma Patterns

Table 4 summarizes the percentage distribution of subject characteristics by longitudinal asthma patterns. Only statistically significant results according to the post-hoc analysis are described.

Table 4. Baseline descriptive characteristics by longitudinal asthma patterns.

	Persistent Asthma Diagnosis with Persistent/Incident Asthma Symptoms (n = 123)	Persistent Asthma Diagnosis with Remittent Asthma Symptoms (n = 21)	Persistent Asthma Symptoms without Asthma Diagnosis (n = 199)	Ex-Asthma (n = 109)	p-Value
Sex (%):					
males	39.0	52.4	52.8	45.9	0.108
females	61.0	47.6	47.2	54.1	
Age (years) (mean ± SD [1])	55.6 ± 16.8	47.9 ± 14.8	61.6 ± 14.1	50.6 ± 13.7	**0.000**
BMI [2] groups (%):					
obese	15.4	4.86	19.1	12.0	**0.000**
overweight	31.7	47.6	43.2	22.2	
underweight/normal weight	52.8	47.6	37.7	65.7	
Educational level (%):					
elementary/junior high school	43.3	23.8	55.8	32.1	**0.000**
high school	37.5	33.3	30.7	44.0	
university	19.2	42.9	13.6	23.9	

[1] SD, standard deviation; [2] BMI, body mass index. Statistically significant values are reported in bold.

Subjects in the pattern "persistent asthma diagnosis with remittent asthma symptoms" showed a younger age and a high educational level; subjects in the pattern "persistent asthma symptoms without asthma diagnosis" exhibited older age, a low educational level and overweight; and "ex-asthma" subjects had a medium educational level and normal weight (Table 4).

3.4. Asthma-Related Indicators by Longitudinal Asthma Patterns

Subjects in the pattern "persistent asthma diagnosis with persistent/incident asthma symptoms" had their first diagnosis and first asthma symptoms at older age with respect to the other asthma patterns (about 26 years of age vs. 9–13 years) and a higher percentage of family history of asthma with respect to those in the pattern "persistent asthma symptoms without asthma diagnosis" (56.1% vs. 32.6%); in addition, subjects in the pattern "persistent asthma diagnosis with persistent/incident asthma symptoms" more frequently reported last 12-month exacerbations (15.6%) (Table 5).

Table 5. Baseline asthma-related indicators by longitudinal asthma patterns.

	Persistent Asthma Diagnosis with Persistent/Incident Asthma Symptoms (n = 123)	Persistent Asthma Diagnosis with Remittent Asthma Symptoms (n = 21)	Persistent Asthma Symptoms without Asthma Diagnosis (n = 199)	Ex-Asthma (n = 109)	p-Value
Age at asthma diagnosis (mean ± SD [1]) [2]	27.1 ± 20.6	9.9 ± 11.6	—	13.8 ± 12.7	**0.000**
Age at first asthma symptoms (mean ± SD [1]) [2]	25.3 ± 20.3	8.0 ± 7.6	—	13.1 ± 12.6	**0.000**
Family history of asthma (%)	56.1	52.4	32.6	35.2	**0.000**
Last 12-month asthma exacerbations [3] (%)	15.6	5.9	4.9	0.0	**0.002**
Last 12-month asthma hospitalizations [3] (%)	5.0	5.9	0.0	1.6	0.144
Last 12-month asthma ED [4] visits [3] (%)	4.2	5.9	1.2	1.6	0.473
Reported SPT [5] positivity (%)	83.5	80.0	65.5	70.5	*0.081*

[1] SD, standard deviation; [2] performed only on subjects reporting lifetime asthma diagnosis; [3] performed only on subjects reporting lifetime asthma diagnosis or symptoms in the last 12 months; [4] ED, emergency department; [5] skin prick test (only subjects performing skin prick test n = 211). Statistically significant values are reported in bold; borderline values are reported in italic.

3.5. Baseline Host and Environmental Risk Factors for Longitudinal Asthma Patterns

Subjects in the pattern "persistent asthma diagnosis with persistent/incident asthma symptoms" showed a higher percentage of asthma comorbidities with respect to the other asthma patterns, except for allergic rhinitis that was higher in the pattern "persistent asthma diagnosis with remittent asthma symptoms" (Table 6).

Table 6. Baseline host and environmental risk factors by longitudinal asthma patterns.

	Persistent Asthma Diagnosis with Persistent/Incident Asthma Symptoms (n = 123)	Persistent Asthma Diagnosis with Remittent Asthma Symptoms (n = 21)	Persistent Asthma Symptoms without Asthma Diagnosis (n = 199)	Ex-Asthma (n = 109)	p-Value
		Asthma comorbidities			
Allergic rhinitis (%)	61.0	66.7	28.3	35.8	**0.000**
GERD [1] (%)	30.1	23.8	34.8	20.6	*0.067*
Sleep apnea (%)	20.3	10.0	18.3	2.8	**0.000**
Recurrent respiratory infections (%)	23.1	4.8	11.3	8.3	**0.003**
COPD [2] (%)	21.1	9.5	11.9	4.6	**0.002**
Nasal polyps	5.7	0.0	4.1	0.0	*0.074*
		Environmental risk factors			
Traffic exposure at home address (%)	69.1	38.1	56.3	54.1	**0.015**
Smoking habits (%): smokers ex-smokers nonsmokers	15.4 34.1 50.4	14.3 28.6 57.1	27.1 47.2 25.6	11.0 36.7 52.3	**0.000**
Secondhand smoke exposure (%)	18.9	9.5	21.4	10.2	*0.066*

[1] GERD, Gastroesophageal reflux disease; [2] COPD, chronic obstructive pulmonary disease. Statistically significant values are reported in bold; borderline values are reported in italic.

Subjects in the pattern "persistent asthma diagnosis with persistent/incident asthma symptoms" showed a higher percentage of traffic exposure at home address and subjects in the pattern "persistent asthma symptoms without asthma diagnosis" a higher percentage of active and passive smoke exposure (Table 6).

Table 7 describes the results of the multinomial logistic regression analysis for the associations among exposures to host and environmental risk factors and longitudinal asthma patterns (with "ex-asthma" as reference category).

Table 7. Factors associated with longitudinal asthma patterns: Odds Ratio and 95% confidence intervals.

	Persistent Asthma Diagnosis with Persistent/Incident Asthma Symptoms	Persistent Asthma Diagnosis with Remittent Asthma Symptoms	Persistent Asthma Symptoms without Asthma Diagnosis
	Host factors		
Allergic rhinitis (ref: no)	**3.12 (1.72–5.69)** 1.00	**3.38 (1.17–9.76)** 1.00	0.99 (0.56–1.78) 1.00
COPD [1] (ref: no)	**4.76 (1.60–4.16)** 1.00	3.48 (0.55–21.94) 1.00	1.32 (0.44–3.97) 1.00
Sleep apnea (ref: no)	**5.99 (1.67–21.39)** 1.00	3.49 (0.50–24.44) 1.00	**5.32 (1.52–18.58)** 1.00
	Environmental factors		
Traffic exposure at home address (ref: no)	**1.86 (1.02–3.38)** 1.00	0.48 (0.17–1.35) 1.00	1.31 (0.75–2.28) 1.00
Smoking habits: smokers ex-smokers (ref: non smokers)	1.59 (0.64–3.96) 0.71 (0.36–1.40) 1.00	1.19 (0.26–5.47) 0.45 (0.13–1.60) 1.00	**6.24 (2.68–14.51)** 1.71 (0.90–3.25) 1.00
Secondhand smoke exposure (ref: no)	**2.64 (1.10–6.33)** 1.00	0.93 (0.17–4.94) 1.00	**3.28 (1.41–7.66)** 1.00
	Adjustment factors		
Age (unit increase)	**1.02 (1.00–1.04)** 1.00	0.98 (0.94–1.02) 1.00	**1.05 (1.03–1.07)** 1.00
Males (ref: females)	0.84 (0.44–1.59) 1.00	1.49 (0.47–4.70) 1.00	0.84 (0.47–1.53) 1.00
BMI categories: obese overweight (ref: underweight/normal weight)	1.46 (0.60–3.51) 1.77 (0.84–3.72) 1.00	0.63 (0.07–5.85) **4.58 (1.33–15.72)** 1.00	1.79 (0.80–4.03) **2.37 (1.20–4.68)** 1.00
Family history of asthma (ref: no)	**2.15 (1.18–3.92)** 1.00	*2.60 (0.91–7.45)* 1.00	0.91 (0.51–1.62) 1.00

[1] COPD, chronic obstructive pulmonary disease; reference category, ex-asthma; in italic, borderline values; in bold, statistically significant values. Adjusted for sex, age, BMI, and family history of asthma.

Allergic rhinitis was significantly associated with a three-fold higher risk of having persistent asthma diagnosis with respect to ex-asthma. COPD was significantly associated with "persistent asthma diagnosis with persistent/incident asthma symptoms" (OR 4.76). Sleep apnea was significantly related to "persistent asthma diagnosis with persistent/incident asthma symptoms" and "persistent asthma symptoms without asthma diagnosis" with a 5–6-fold higher risk (Table 7).

Concerning the environmental factors, traffic exposure near home was significantly related to "persistent asthma diagnosis with persistent/incident asthma symptoms" (OR 1.86) and active smoke to "persistent asthma symptoms without asthma diagnosis" (OR 6.24). Passive smoke was significantly associated with "persistent asthma diagnosis with persistent/incident asthma symptoms" and "persistent asthma symptoms without asthma diagnosis" with a 2.6–3.3-fold higher risk (Table 7).

Finally, significant associations were found among: increasing age and higher risk of having asthma symptoms (with/without diagnosis); overweight and a 4.6- and 2.4-fold higher risk of having "persistent asthma diagnosis with remittent asthma symptoms" and "persistent asthma symptoms without asthma diagnosis", respectively; and family history of asthma and higher risk of "persistent asthma diagnosis with persistent/incident asthma symptoms" (OR 2.15) (Table 7).

4. Discussion

Using an unsupervised approach (LTA), we detected four main longitudinal asthma patterns in a sample of adult general population: "persistent asthma diagnosis with persistent/incident asthma symptoms" (27.2%), "persistent asthma diagnosis with remittent asthma symptoms" (4.6%), "persistent asthma symptoms without asthma diagnosis" (44.0%), and "ex-asthma" (24.1%). These patterns were related to different host and environmental risk factors.

4.1. Comorbidities

Subjects with allergic rhinitis had a three-fold significantly higher risk of having persistent asthma diagnosis with respect to "exasthma", highlighting the importance of active management of allergic comorbidities in asthma patients because they may contribute to symptoms burden and poor asthma control, as reported by the international guidelines [1]. Asthma and allergic rhinitis share a similar inflammatory process and nasal allergen exposure in patients with allergic rhinitis yields a generalized airway inflammation including lower airways [1,10].

"Persistent asthma diagnosis with persistent/incident asthma symptoms" was significantly related to COPD (OR 4.76). Asthma and COPD are strongly related, even if they are heterogeneous diseases with various underlying mechanisms. There is broad agreement that patients with features of both diseases have frequent exacerbations, poor quality of life and a more rapid decline in lung function and high mortality [1]. In a US general adult population sample (≥65 years) with active asthma, patients with COPD had a four-fold higher risk of having asthma-related hospitalizations in the last 12 months [26]. A similar result was found in a Canadian study, using health administrative databases: higher rates of asthma claims were found in patients with than in those without COPD [27]. Moreover, active asthma was significantly associated with an increased risk for chronic bronchitis, emphysema, and COPD over a 20-year follow-up [28].

Sleep apnea was significantly related to "persistent asthma diagnosis with persistent/incident asthma symptoms" and "persistent asthma symptoms without asthma diagnosis" with a 5–6-fold higher risk (OR 5.99 and OR 5.32, respectively). Asthma and sleep apnea share many predisposing and aggravating factors; asthma is often accompanied by snoring and apnea, and sleep apnea often combines with asthma. The two diseases present many similar features [29,30] and recent studies have shown that asthma and sleep apnea share a bidirectional relationship where each disorder adversely influences the other one [30,31]. As reported in a US study, unrecognized sleep apnea could be a reason for persistent asthma symptoms during the day and the night [32]. On the other side, the presence of a diagnosed disease with similar clinical manifestations, such as sleep apnea, might lead to lack of recognition or misinterpretation of asthma symptoms, justifying the strong relationship found with persistent asthma symptoms without lifetime asthma diagnosis [29].

4.2. Environmental Risk Factors

Reported traffic exposure near home was significantly associated with "persistent asthma diagnosis with persistent/incident asthma symptoms" (OR 1.86 vs. "ex-asthma"). Urban living, characterized by high concentration of air pollutants emitted by vehicular traffic, is an important risk factor for asthma onset and exacerbations [33–35]. Recent studies showed a higher risk of persistent asthma in ≥45-year-old subjects living <200 m from a major road (OR 5.21) [36] and a higher risk of last 12-month asthma attacks (OR 1.35) or wheezing (OR 1.24) in adult subjects exposed to moderate/heavy traffic near home [37]. Moreover, the current data are in line with our previous observations that urban living, with respect to rural living, is associated with several adverse effects: e.g., larger prevalence of respiratory symptoms/diseases [17] and higher bronchial hyper-responsiveness, which is an important marker of active asthma [38].

A significantly higher risk of "persistent asthma symptoms without asthma diagnosis" was found in current smokers (OR 6.24), which might indicate underdiagnosis of asthma in this group [39,40].

This relationship emerged also in UK and US studies where active smoke was a risk factor for undiagnosed wheeze at 18 years old (OR 2.54 and OR 2.60, respectively) [39,41]. In a recent paper about the same UK sample, subjects identified as "undiagnosed-wheezers" phenotype had the highest prevalence of smoking habit (74.6%) with respect to the other "wheezers" phenotypes [42]. A possible explanation is that respiratory symptoms, such as wheeze or breathlessness, are misinterpreted as due to smoking, rather than referred to asthmatic condition and, thus, not reported to the physician. On the other hand, asthma-like symptoms are also common in subjects with COPD, which is often smoke-related, making it difficult to disentangle the relationship between smoking and asthma-like symptoms. Smoking plays an important role in asthma management, since asthmatic smokers have worse clinical outcomes compared with nonsmokers, i.e., increased morbidity and mortality, higher frequency of exacerbations, reduced lung function, and worse quality of life [43,44].

Finally, in our study, a strong relationship was found between "persistent asthma diagnosis with persistent/incident asthma symptoms" or "persistent asthma symptoms without asthma diagnosis" and secondhand smoke (OR 2.64 and OR 3.28, respectively). Respiratory health effects of involuntary smoking among children/adolescents are well documented, but fewer studies took into account adult subjects. A study performed on an Italian sample of nonsmoker women showed that passive smoke exposure both to husband and at work resulted a significant risk factor for asthma symptoms (OR 1.71 for recent wheeze and OR 1.85 for recent attacks of shortness of breath with wheeze) [45]. Similar results were found in a Danish study on an adult sample showing that persons exposed to passive smoke were at increased risk of wheeze (OR 1.69) and decreased lung function [46].

4.3. Limitations and Strengths

A limitation of this study is the use of a questionnaire for collecting data on respiratory symptoms/diseases, potentially affected by a reporting bias, as it relies upon individual memory. Thus, the estimates of "underdiagnosed" asthma (persistent asthma symptoms without lifetime diagnosis) might be biased, particularly in older subjects, because elderly people with an early onset of the disease may more frequently forget that they had a physician diagnosis, differently from younger people with a more reliable recall. As a consequence, this differential recall bias might have affected the estimates of the time trends and the assessment of the determinants of asthma patterns [47]. Nevertheless, the standardized questionnaire is one of the main investigation tools in respiratory epidemiology [48] and our questions were derived from validated international questionnaires, which already had passed the scrutiny of independent reviewers.

A participation rate of 68% was obtained in the AGAVE study. Comparing the characteristics of subjects included in the AGAVE survey vs. those lost to follow-up, few differences were found, with a lower mean age and more females in the AGAVE sample. No difference was found when considering the enrollment criteria (percentage of asthma symptoms and/or diagnosis in the previous surveys). Moreover, the same cross-sectional asthma phenotypes that emerged in the AGAVE survey were found in the previous surveys, although with different proportions (Table S1). Thus, the AGAVE sample can be considered representative of the previous samples from which it was extracted according to the enrollment criteria.

The strength of our study is to have analyzed risk factors related to adult asthma patterns in a real-life setting using a multidimensional and unsupervised data analysis approach (the latent transition analysis) which has the advantage of being free from a priori assumptions. Indeed, the choice of the variables to be included in the model was warranted by their clinical relevance, representing the main dimensions of asthma, even if the choice is subjective and may condition the obtained classes [49].

LTA provides innovative perspectives to epidemiological studies. Indeed, while the standard approaches focus on true dichotomous outcomes (disease present or absent), LTA focus on the concept of phenotype, i.e., a combination of several clinical presentations that may occur or not with a given probability. Moreover, LTA is able to describe phenotype changes over time [14].

Finally, it is worth mentioning that a follow-up of these patients will be performed in a new project, starting in the next months, in order to assess the clinical meaning of the detected phenotypes and their relevance for disease prognosis, with special focus on the multimorbidity condition.

5. Conclusions

This study about adult asthmatic cohort showed that asthma patterns were differently associated with comorbidities and environmental risk factors exposure. It highlights the necessity of a careful monitoring of exposure to active and passive smoke and to vehicular traffic near the house of residence in the general population, which are possible determinants of occurrence of asthma symptoms (with or without lifetime diagnosis). The increased awareness of these relevant factors and the inclusion of such information in current guidelines could be useful to patients and healthcare providers in prevention and management strategies.

Supplementary Materials: The following are available online at http://www.mdpi.com/2077-0383/9/11/3632/s1, Table S1: Comparison among AGAVE and previous-surveys cross-sectional phenotypes (%); Supplementary S1: Extract from the AGAVE questionnaire.

Author Contributions: Conceptualization, S.M., S.B., A.A. and G.V.; Data curation, S.B., M.S. and A.A.; Formal analysis, S.M. and S.F.; Funding acquisition, G.V.; Investigation, S.B., M.S. and A.A.; Methodology, S.F.; Supervision, G.V.; Writing—original draft, S.M.; and Writing—review and editing, S.M., S.B., S.L.G., V.M., S.F. and G.V. All authors have read and agreed to the published version of the manuscript.

Funding: This work was supported in part by the CNR-ENEL (Italian Electric Power Authority) "Interaction of Energy Systems with Human Health and Environment" Project (1989), the Italian National Research Council Targeted Project "Prevention and Control Disease Factors-SP 2"(Contract No. 91.00171.PF41; 1991), and the Italian Medicines Agency (AIFA), within the independent drug research program (Contract No. FARM8YRYZC; 2010).

Conflicts of Interest: The authors declare no conflict of interest. The funders had no role in the design of the study; in the collection, analyses, or interpretation of data; in the writing of the manuscript, or in the decision to publish the results.

References

1. Global Initiative for Asthma. Global Strategy for Asthma Management and Prevention. Update Accessed January, 2019. Available online: https://ginasthma.org/2018-gina-report-global-strategy-for-asthma-management-and-prevention/ (accessed on 18 September 2020).
2. Maio, S.; Baldacci, S.; Simoni, M.; Angino, A.; Martini, F.; Cerrai, S.; Sarno, G.; Pala, A.; Bresciani, M.; ARGA Study Group; et al. Impact of Asthma and Comorbid Allergic Rhinitis on Quality of Life and Control in Patients of Italian General Practitioners. *J. Asthma* **2012**, *49*, 854–861. [CrossRef] [PubMed]
3. Von Mutius, E.; Smits, H.H. Primary prevention of asthma: From risk and protective factors to targeted strategies for prevention. *Lancet* **2020**. [CrossRef]
4. GBD 2017 Causes of Death Collaborators. Global, regional, and national age-sex-specific mortality for 282 causes of death in 195 countries and territories, 1980–2017: A systematic analysis for the Global Burden of Disease Study. *Lancet* **2018**, *392*, 1736–1788. [CrossRef]
5. James, S.L.; Abate, D.; Abate, K.H.; Abay, S.M.; Abbafati, C.; Abbasi, N.; Abbastabar, H.; Abd-Allah, F.; Abdela, J.; Abdelalim, A.; et al. GBD 2017 Disease and Injury Incidence and Prevalence Collaborators: Global, regional, and national incidence, prevalence, and years lived with disability for 354 diseases and injuries for 195 countries and territories, 1990–2017: A systematic analysis for the Global Burden of Disease Study. *Lancet* **2018**, *392*, 1789–1858. [CrossRef]
6. Guerra, S. Clinical remission of asthma: What lies beyond? *Thorax* **2005**, *60*, 5–6. [CrossRef]
7. Gershon, A.; Guan, J.; Victor, J.; Wang, C.; To, T. The course of asthma activity: A population study. *J. Allergy Clin. Immunol.* **2012**, *129*, 679–686. [CrossRef]
8. Trivedi, M.; Denton, E. Asthma in Children and Adults—What Are the Differences and What Can They Tell us about Asthma? *Front. Pediatr.* **2019**, *7*, 256. [CrossRef]

9. To, M.; Tsuzuki, R.; Katsube, O.; Yamawaki, S.; Soeda, S.; Kono, Y.; Honda, N.; Kano, I.; Haruki, K.; To, Y. Persistent Asthma from Childhood to Adulthood Presents a Distinct Phenotype of Adult Asthma. *J. Allergy Clin. Immunol. Pract.* **2020**, *8*, 1921–1927. [CrossRef]
10. Yavuz, S.T.; Civelek, E.; Comert, S.; Sahiner, U.M.; Buyuktiryaki, B.; Tuncer, A.; Kalyoncu, A.F.; Sekerel, B.E. Development of rhinitis may be an indicator for the persistence of childhood asthma. *Int. J. Pediatr. Otorhinolaryngol.* **2014**, *78*, 843–849. [CrossRef]
11. Papaioannou, A.I.; Kostikas, K.; Zervas, E.; Kolilekas, L.; Papiris, S.; Gaga, M. Control of asthma in real life: Still a valuable goal? *Eur. Respir. Rev.* **2015**, *24*, 361–369. [CrossRef]
12. Garden, F.L.; Simpson, J.M.; Mellis, C.M.; Marks, G.B. For the CAPS Investigator. Change in the manifestations of asthma and asthma-related traits in childhood: A latent transition analysis. *Eur. Respir. J.* **2016**, *47*, 499–509. [CrossRef] [PubMed]
13. Brew, B.K.; Chiesa, F.; Lundholm, C.; Örtqvist, A.; Almqvist, C. A modern approach to identifying and characterizing child asthma and wheeze phenotypes based on clinical data. *PLoS ONE* **2019**, *14*, e0227091. [CrossRef] [PubMed]
14. Soto-Ramírez, N.; Ziyab, A.H.; Karmaus, W.; Zhang, H.; Kurukulaaratchy, R.J.; Ewart, S.; Arshad, S.H. Epidemiologic Methods of Assessing Asthma and Wheezing Episodes in Longitudinal Studies: Measures of Change and Stability. *J. Epidemiol.* **2013**, *23*, 399–410. [CrossRef] [PubMed]
15. Amaral, R.; Pereira, A.M.; Jacinto, T.; Malinovschi, A.; Janson, C.; Alving, K.; Fonseca, J.A. Comparison of hypothesis- and data-driven asthma phenotypes in NHANES 2007–2012: The importance of comprehensive data availability. *Clin. Transl. Allergy* **2019**, *9*, 17. [CrossRef] [PubMed]
16. Maio, S.; Baldacci, S.; Bresciani, M.; Simoni, M.; Latorre, M.; Murgia, N.; Spinozzi, F.; Braschi, M.; Antonicelli, L.; Brunetto, B.; et al. RItA: The Italian severe/uncontrolled asthma registry. *Allergy* **2018**, *73*, 683–695. [CrossRef]
17. Viegi, G.; Pedreschi, M.; Baldacci, S.; Chiaffi, L.; Pistelli, F.; Modena, P.; Vellutini, M.; Di Pede, F.; Carrozzi, L. Prevalence rates of respiratory symptoms and diseases in general population samples of North and Central Italy. *Int. J. Tuberc. Lung Dis.* **1999**, *3*, 1034–1042.
18. Maio, S.; Baldacci, S.; Carrozzi, L.; Pistelli, F.; Angino, A.; Simoni, M.; Sarno, G.; Cerrai, S.; Martini, F.; Fresta, M.; et al. Respiratory symptoms/diseases prevalence is still increasing: A 25-yr population study. *Respir. Med.* **2016**, *110*, 58–68. [CrossRef]
19. The European Community Respiratory Health Survey II Steering Committee. The European Community Respiratory Health Survey II. *Eur. Respir. J.* **2002**, *20*, 1071–1079. [CrossRef]
20. Fazzi, P.; Viegi, G.; Paoletti, P.; Giuliano, G.; Begliomini, E.; Fornai, E.; Giuntini, C. Comparison between two standardized questionnaires in a group of workers. *Eur. J. Respir. Dis.* **1982**, *63*, 168–169.
21. Viegi, G.; Paoletti, P.; Prediletto, R.; Carrozzi, L.; Fazzi, P.; Di Pede, F.; Pistelli, G.; Giuntini, C.; Lebowitz, M.D. Prevalence of respiratory symptoms in an unpolluted area of northern Italy. *Eur. Respir. J.* **1988**, *1*, 311–318.
22. Viegi, G. Indicators and biological mechanisms of impairment of the respiratory system by environmental pollutants. An operational example: Epidemiological studies of the delta of Po and the region of Pisa. *Epidemiol. Prev.* **1995**, *19*, 66–75. [PubMed]
23. Weinmayr, G.; Keller, F.; Kleiner, A.; du Prel, J.B.; Garcia-Marcos, L.; Batllés-Garrido, J.; Garcia-Hernandez, G.; Suarez-Varela, M.M.; Strachan, D.P.; Nagel, G. Asthma phenotypes identified by latent class analysis in the ISAAC phase II Spain study. *Clin. Exp. Allergy* **2013**, *43*, 223–232. [CrossRef] [PubMed]
24. Boudier, A.; Curjuric, I.; Basagaña, X.; Hazgui, H.; Anto, J.M.; Bousquet, J.; Bridevaux, P.O.; Dupuis-Lozeron, E.; Garcia-Aymerich, J.; Heinrich, J.; et al. Ten-Year Follow-up of Cluster-based Asthma Phenotypes in Adults. A Pooled Analysis of Three Cohorts. *Am. J. Respir. Crit. Care Med.* **2013**, *188*, 550–560. [CrossRef] [PubMed]
25. Collins, L.M.; Lanza, S.T. *Latent Class and Latent Transition Analysis with Applications in the Social, Behavioral, and Health Sciences*; Wiley Series in Probability and Statistics 2010; Balding, D., Cressie, N.A.C., Fitzmaurice, G.M., Johnstone, I.M., Molenberghs, G., Scott, L., Smith, A.F.M., Tsay, R.S., Weisberg, S.P., Eds.; A John Wiley & Sons, Inc.: Hoboken, NJ, USA, 2010; pp. 1–283.
26. Hsu, J.; Chen, J.; Mirabelli, M.C. Asthma Morbidity, Comorbidities, and Modifiable Factors among Older Adults. *J. Allergy Clin. Immunol. Pract.* **2018**, *6*, 236–243. [CrossRef] [PubMed]
27. Anderson, H.M.; Jackson, D.J. Microbes, allergic sensitization, and the natural history of asthma. *Curr. Opin. Allergy Clin. Immunol.* **2017**, *17*, 116–122. [CrossRef] [PubMed]
28. Silva, G.E.; Sherrill, D.L.; Guerra, S.; Barbee, R.A. Asthma as a risk factor for COPD in a longitudinal study. *Chest* **2004**, *126*, 59–65. [CrossRef] [PubMed]

29. Qiao, Y.-X.; Xiao, Y. Asthma and Obstructive Sleep Apnea. *Chin. Med. J.* **2015**, *128*, 2798–2804. [CrossRef]
30. Prasad, B.; Nyenhuis, S.M.; Imayama, I.; Siddiqi, A.; Teodorescu, M. Asthma and Obstructive Sleep Apnea Overlap: What Has the Evidence Taught Us? *Am. J. Respir. Crit. Care Med.* **2020**, *201*, 1345–1357. [CrossRef]
31. Dixit, R.; Verma, S.; Gupta, N.; Sharma, A.; Chandran, A. Obstructive Sleep Apnea in Bronchial Asthma Patients: Assessment of Prevalence and Risk Factors. *J. Assoc. Physicians India* **2018**, *66*, 45–48.
32. Teodorescu, M.; Polomis, D.A.; Teodorescu, M.C.; Gangnon, R.E.; Peterson, A.G.; Consens, F.B.; Chervin, R.D.; Jarjour, N.N. Association of obstructive sleep apnea risk or diagnosis with daytime asthma in adults. *J. Asthma* **2012**, *49*, 620–628. [CrossRef]
33. Prüss-Üstün, A.; Wolf, J.; Corvalán, C.; Bos, R.; Neira, M. Preventing Disease through Healthy Environments. A Global Assessment of the Burden of Disease from Environmental Risks. WHO. 2016. Available online: http://www.who.int/quantifying_ehimpacts/publications/preventing-disease/en/ (accessed on 18 September 2020).
34. Thurston, G.D.; Kipen, H.; Annesi-Maesano, I.; Balmes, J.; Brook, R.D.; Cromar, K.; De Matteis, S.; Forastiere, F.; Forsberg, B.; Frampton, M.W.; et al. A joint ERS/ATS policy statement: What constitutes an adverse health effect of air pollution? An analytical framework. *Eur. Respir. J.* **2017**, *49*, 1600419. [CrossRef] [PubMed]
35. Thurston, G.D.; Balmes, J.R.; Garcia, E.; Gilliland, F.D.; Rice, M.B.; Schikowski, T.; Van Winkle, L.S.; Annesi-Maesano, I.; Burchard, E.G.; Carlsten, C.; et al. Outdoor Air Pollution and New-Onset Airway Disease. An Official American Thoracic Society Workshop Report. *Ann. Am. Thorac. Soc.* **2020**, *17*, 387–398. [CrossRef] [PubMed]
36. Bowatte, G.; Lodge, C.J.; Knibbs, L.D.; Erbas, B.; Perret, J.L.; Jalaludin, B.; Morgan, G.G.; Bui, D.S.; Giles, G.G.; Hamilton, G.S.; et al. Traffic related air pollution and development and persistence of asthma and low lung function. *Environ. Int.* **2018**, *113*, 170–176. [CrossRef] [PubMed]
37. Hegseth, M.N.; Oftedal, B.M.; Höper, A.C.; Aminoff, A.L.; Thomassen, M.R.; Svendsen, M.V.; Fell, A.K.M. Self-reported traffic-related air pollution and respiratory symptoms among adults in an area with modest levels of traffic. *PLoS ONE* **2019**, *14*, e0226221. [CrossRef] [PubMed]
38. Maio, S.; Baldacci, S.; Carrozzi, L.; Polverino, E.; Angino, A.; Pistelli, F.; Di Pede, F.; Simoni, M.; Sherrill, D.; Viegi, G. Urban residence is associated with bronchial hyperresponsiveness in Italian general population samples. *Chest* **2009**, *135*, 434–441. [CrossRef]
39. Raza, A.; Kurukulaaratchy, R.J.; Grundy, J.D.; Clayton, C.B.; Mitchell, F.A.; Roberts, G.; Ewart, S.; Sadeghnejad, A.; Arshad, S.H. What does adolescent undiagnosed wheeze represent? Findings from the Isle of Wight Cohort. *Eur. Respir. J.* **2012**, *40*, 580–588. [CrossRef]
40. Accordini, S.; Cappa, V.; Braggion, M.; Corsico, A.G.; Bugiani, M.; Pirina, P.; Verlato, G.; Villani, S.; de Marco, R. The impact of diagnosed and undiagnosed current asthma in the general adult population. *Int. Arch. Allergy Immunol.* **2011**, *155*, 403–411. [CrossRef]
41. Yeatts, K.; Davis, K.J.; Sotir, M.; Herget, C.; Shy, C. Who gets diagnosed with asthma? Frequent wheeze among adolescents with and without a diagnosis of asthma. *Pediatrics* **2003**, *111*, 1046–1054. [CrossRef]
42. Kurukulaaratchy, R.J.; Zhang, H.; Raza, A.; Patil, V.; Karmaus, W.; Ewart, S.; Arshad, S.H. The Diversity of Young Adult Wheeze; a Cluster Analysis in a Longitudinal Birth Cohort. *Clin. Exp. Allergy* **2014**, *44*, 724–735. [CrossRef]
43. Thomson, N.C. Asthma and smoking-induced airway disease without spirometric COPD. *Eur. Respir. J.* **2017**, *49*, 1602061. [CrossRef]
44. Chatkin, J.M.; Dullius, C.R. The management of asthmatic smokers. *Asthma Res. Pract.* **2016**, *2*, 10. [CrossRef] [PubMed]
45. Simoni, M.; Baldacci, S.; Puntoni, R.; Pistelli, F.; Farchi, S.; Lo Presti, E.; Pistelli, R.; Corbo, G.; Agabiti, N.; Basso, S.; et al. Respiratory symptoms/diseases and environmental tobacco smoke (ETS) in never smoker Italian women. *Respir. Med.* **2007**, *101*, 531–538. [CrossRef] [PubMed]
46. Hersoug, L.G.; Husemoen, L.L.; Sigsgaard, T.; Madsen, F.; Linneberg, A. Indoor exposure to environmental cigarette smoke, but not other inhaled particulates associates with respiratory symptoms and diminished lung function in adults. *Respirology* **2010**, *15*, 993–1000. [CrossRef]
47. Pesce, G.; Locatelli, F.; Cerveri, I.; Bugiani, M.; Pirina, P.; Johannessen, A.; Accordini, S.; Zanolin, M.E.; Verlato, G.; de Marco, R. Seventy Years of Asthma in Italy: Age, Period and Cohort Effects on Incidence and Remission of Self-Reported Asthma from 1940 to 2010. *PLoS ONE* **2015**, *10*, e0138570. [CrossRef] [PubMed]

48. Pistelli, F.; Maio, S. Questionnaires and lung function. In *Respiratory Epidemiology*; Annesi-Maesano, I., Lundback, B., Viegi, G., Eds.; European Respiratory Society Publications: Sheffield, UK, 2014; Volume 65, pp. 257–272.
49. Bougas, N.; Just, J.; Beydon, N.; De Blic, J.; Gabet, S.; Lezmi, G.; Amat, F.; Rancière, F.; Momas, I. Unsupervised trajectories of respiratory/allergic symptoms throughout childhood in the PARIS cohort. *Pediatr. Allergy Immunol.* **2019**, *30*, 315–324. [CrossRef] [PubMed]

Publisher's Note: MDPI stays neutral with regard to jurisdictional claims in published maps and institutional affiliations.

© 2020 by the authors. Licensee MDPI, Basel, Switzerland. This article is an open access article distributed under the terms and conditions of the Creative Commons Attribution (CC BY) license (http://creativecommons.org/licenses/by/4.0/).

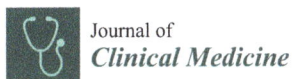

Review

Diet: A Specific Part of the Western Lifestyle Pack in the Asthma Epidemic

Carmen Frontela-Saseta [1,2,*], Carlos A. González-Bermúdez [2] and Luis García-Marcos [2]

1. Department of Food Science and Nutrition, Faculty of Veterinary Sciences, Regional Campus of International Excellence "Campus Mare Nostrum", 30100 Murcia, Spain
2. Biomedical Research Institute of Murcia (IMIB-Arrixaca), University of Murcia, 30003 Murcia, Spain; cagb1@um.es (C.A.G.-B.); lgmarcos@um.es (L.G.-M.)
* Correspondence: carmenfr@um.es

Received: 24 May 2020; Accepted: 27 June 2020; Published: 1 July 2020

Abstract: The Western lifestyle is a complex concept that includes the diet as the main axis of different factors which contribute to a detrimental effect on health, lower life expectancy and low quality-of-life. This type of diet is characterized by being high in calories, mainly provided by saturated fats, and rich in sugars that can lead to changes in immune cells and their responsiveness, by different mechanisms that have yet to be totally clarified. Inflammatory processes are perpetuated through different pathways, in which adipose tissue is a major factor. High fat stores in overweight and obesity accumulate energy but the endocrine function is also producing and releasing different bioactive compounds, adipokines, known to be pro-inflammatory and which play an important role in the pathogenesis of asthma. This review therefore explores the latest evidence regarding the adverse effect of the Western diet on adipose tissue inflammation and its causative effect on the asthma epidemic.

Keywords: Western lifestyle; saturated fats; simple carbohydrates; obesity; adipose tissue; inflammation; asthma

1. Introduction

Inflammatory diseases are increasing worldwide to epidemic proportions and are considered lifestyle-associated diseases, similar to obesity [1]. These pathologies have a multifactorial cause in which diet is a well-known environmental factor involved in obesity, whilst in the etiology of other inflammatory diseases, diet is gaining increasing attention as a risk factor. With regard to this, the Western diet is characterized, broadly speaking, by a high content of saturated fats and simple sugars and a low content of plant-origin foods, and is associated with an increased risk of inflammatory diseases, including asthma.

This kind of diet usually includes foods rich in calories and their regular consumption can lead to overweight and obesity, which basically consists of an excess of body-fat stores. This adipose tissue seems to be an important factor in systemic inflammation, including airway inflammation (asthma), and especially in the case of obesity, which is characterized by excessive accumulation of fat [2]. From this perspective, this review examines the evidence for the association between asthma and nutrition, and specifically addresses the effect of Western diets on the inflammatory processes, reviewing the causative relationships with the adipose tissue.

2. Diet and the Parallel Epidemics of Obesity and Asthma

There is a growing body of evidence on the association between asthma and nutrition. Although the exact mechanisms of this association are far from clear, the epidemiological data suggest that this is indeed the case.

From the most elemental point of view, there has been a parallel increase between the asthma and the obesity epidemics [3], with the latter being closely related to changes in nutrition [4]. According to the epidemiological data on asthma tracking back to the 1960s and 1970s [5–7], in the Nordic and English-speaking countries, there has been an increase in asthma prevalence in all age groups. That same trend has been found in Mediterranean countries [8]. Those regional reports were later supported, albeit partially, by the findings from the International Study of Asthma and Allergies in Childhood (ISAAC), which compared prevalence data from its Phases One (carried out between 1994 and 1995) and Three (performed between 2002 and 2003) [9]. There was, however, a different note here as the authors suggested that the prevalence had increased among both schoolchildren as well as adolescents in those countries where the asthma prevalence had previously been lower, while it was stable or even reduced in countries with a formerly higher prevalence.

The obesity epidemic, which relates to nutrition and sedentarism, tracks back to similar years to that of asthma and shows a parallel increasing trend starting at a higher prevalence [3]. This does not necessarily mean that the two epidemics really started at the same time, but the epidemiological data available track back in an interesting parallel way. Curiously, a similar behavior to the asthma epidemic seems to be happening at least in some populations: both in adults and adolescents, the rise in prevalence occurring from the 1970s seems to have slowed down or even halted [10,11].

Taking this phenomenon into consideration, whether nutrition disorders lead to obesity and this to asthma (through altering lung mechanics, for instance), or asthma favors obesity (through sedentarism, for example), or asthma and obesity are effects of common parallel causes (including nutrition) is a matter of certain debate and is probably dependent upon each individual.

There are certain facts that relate obesity to asthma, starting from a common genetic predisposition, as shown by studies in twins. The study by Hallstrand et al., including 1001 monozygotic and 383 dizygotic twin pairs of the same sex, arrived at the conclusion that apart from there being a strong association between asthma and body mass index (BMI), there was also an important heritability for asthma (53%) and obesity (77%) with additive genetic influences in each condition [12]. However, a second study from the Danish Twin Registry [13], including 29,183 twin individuals, found that the heritability of obesity was higher (81% in males and 92% in females) as was that of asthma (78% and 68%, respectively). However, their analyses of age-adjusted genetic liabilities to asthma and obesity were significantly correlated only in females, and this was related to common genes.

Nevertheless, diet has been shown to be independently associated to asthma at the epidemiological level. For instance, in cross-sectional studies, a Mediterranean diet has been shown to be associated to a lower prevalence of asthma, independently of BMI [14,15], whilst frequent fast-food consumption seems to be a risk factor for asthma [16]. Furthermore, the frequent consumption of anti-oxidant foods has been associated to lower asthma prevalence [17,18]. Those dietary profiles (Mediterranean diet versus fast food) also have important implications for obesity. On the other hand, the frequent consumption (three or more times per week versus never or occasionally) of individual foods such as fruit and vegetables have been related to lower BMI and to lower asthma prevalence in adolescents worldwide [16,19].

More interestingly, the influence of certain factors related to both asthma and obesity seem to be important during pregnancy or during the first weeks of life. For instance, adherence to a Mediterranean diet by the mother in pregnancy seems to have implications for both asthma and obesity [20]. Moreover, maternal obesity in pregnancy is associated to both asthma and obesity in the offspring [21,22].

Thus, it is quite probable that nutrition influences obesity and asthma in parallel, independently of the interaction of the two conditions on each other, no matter whether the mechanisms of this interaction are purely mechanic, inflammatory, or others, and this influence occurs more easily in genetically predisposed individuals. The purpose of this review is to summarize the current evidence on the connections between nutrients highly present in the Western diet and asthma, as well as the possible mechanisms involved.

2.1. Role of Micronutrients and Macronutrients

The relationship between environmental factors, such as diet, and asthma risk is very complex and thus not fully understood [23]. The effects of individual nutrients on health have been widely studied in order to better understand the effects of isolated compounds on different diseases. However, nowadays, the study of specific dietary patterns and foods as complex matrices and their effect on health and disease prevention is gaining attention [24]. Regarding this, diets rich in vegetables are clearly related with valuable effects in preventing different diseases, whilst diets rich in calories, and overall when that energy is mainly provided by fat-rich foods, are strongly linked with chronic inflammatory processes, such as asthma, among others [25]. These fat-rich foods, usually consumed as part of the Western-style dietary patterns which are also considered as obesogenic, are often associated to an increased access to highly processed foods that are related with high contents of simple sugars and saturated fats and low contents of minerals and vitamins [26]. It is clear that this change in dietary patterns modifies general diet quality, which is involved in the development of different diseases, mainly those related with inflammation, cardiovascular risk, aging process [27], and also with the increasing burden of asthma [28], mainly through the control of various immune pathways; specifically, with the role of macro- and micro-nutrients on them being clearly different.

This type of pattern (Western diet) also includes reduced intake of micronutrients (vitamins and minerals), dietary fiber, unsaturated fatty acids and a low consumption of a wide variety of bioactive compounds that, in isolation, have been reported as having different interesting beneficial properties [29], and when they are consumed as part of a diet, may act together with more favorable effects on health status and disease management, including asthma [30]. Furthermore, typical Western foods are usually poor in fiber, providing daily amounts below the recommended 30 g, which is correlated with a higher risk of respiratory diseases related with an increase in short chain fatty acids' (SCFA) production in the colon, which are systemically distributed [31].

Within the dietary foodstuffs included in the Mediterranean diet, fish consumption is highly recommended and implies the intake of fatty acids with a predominance of the w-3 profile that are able to partly inhibit a number of aspects of inflammation [32] and have been proposed as protective metabolites for asthma. However, this effect has been demonstrated when marine oil is abundantly consumed in the diet, provided by one serving of fish per day. This, although it can be obtained through the diet, is not a usual habit. Based on this, including 2–3 portions per week of sardines, mackerel, herring, tuna or salmon in addition to foods rich in different compounds with anti-inflammatory activity, such as those included in the Mediterranean diet, would help to achieve sufficient amounts of bioactive compounds to reduce inflammatory pathways.

The increased distance from this dietary pattern has alarmingly increased overweight and obesity, as well as related diseases, in recent years [33]. In obesity, excessive weight gain leads to adipose tissue remodeling, adipocyte hypertrophy, hypoxia, stress and apoptosis/necrosis, including a prolonged production of inflammatory mediators, with the subsequent release of adipose-derived pro-inflammatory cytokines and free fatty acids into the circulation. This can lead to systemic disturbances in metabolism and tissue health, promoting chronic low-grade inflammation and an increased risk for chronic diseases [34]. With regard to this, it has recently been reported that fat mass loss compared to BMI or weight can further improve different risk profiles and inflammation-related biomarkers and also shows a high capability for predicting the cardiometabolic profile [35]. This highlights the importance of body fat in the inflammatory response and how the accumulation of excessive fat, as in the case of obesity, may interfere with the maintenance of an optimal state of health [2]. Inflammatory mediators are stimulated by macronutrients in the adipose tissues that are mainly incorporated as flux through the diet as carbohydrates and fats that, after absorption, are stored in adipose tissue. It is important to highlight that not only the total amount of calories consumed but also their distribution, mainly across fats and/or carbohydrates, have a different impact on adipose tissue and thus on the incidence/severity of asthma [2,36].

Overconsumption of macronutrients in the diet stimulates the adipose tissue to release inflammatory mediators, predisposing the pro-inflammatory state in addition to increasing the risk and severity of infections [37,38]; moreover, micronutrient deficiencies (especially regarding those which are lipophilic: vitamins A, D, E, K and carotenoids) have a negative impact on the regulation of adipose tissue biology with respect to the modulation of adipogenesis or inflammatory status that gain importance related with obesity and associated pathologies. Regarding this, there is also information indicating that diet composition (the type of dietary macro- and micro-nutrients), independently of its caloric content, can influence the function of adipose tissue in different ways and the expression and secretion of inflammatory biomarkers [37].

In this way, complex dietary carbohydrates (starches, glucans, fructans and cellulose), and especially those from whole-grain products, have demonstrated an inverse association with inflammation and adipose tissue deposition but also depending on the gut microbiota population [38]. Meanwhile, elevated simple carbohydrates' (sugars mainly used as sweeteners, such as glucose and fructose) consumption promotes the inflammatory state and acts on adipose tissue, inducing lipogenesis, because, in excess, they are converted into fatty acids, mainly palmitate, and promote lipid synthesis. Simple carbohydrates are highly consumed in the Western diet, and based on their effects on health, we can affirm that limiting the consumption of simple/refined grains and increasing the intake of whole grains is highly recommended [39]. Moreover, the high consumption of simple sugars used as sweeteners in different sugary beverages, that are widely consumed in this kind of diet, has been associated with asthma being more evident in case of beverages containing a high fructose:glucose ratio that can cause fructose malabsorption, resulting in the intestinal formation of pro-inflammatory products between unabsorbed fructose and some dietary proteins that, after intestinal absorption, are associated with asthma [40].

Focusing on dietary fats, they are mainly consumed as triglycerides and great differences and biological effects on tissues can be found, depending on the type of fatty acid after lipolysis. An increase in the intake of monounsaturated fatty acids (MUFAs) (mainly oleic acid, abundant in olive oil), omega-3 polyunsaturated fatty acids (PUFAs) (alpha linolenic acid, abundant in seeds and vegetables, and eicosapentanoic (EPA) and docosahexanoic (DHA) acids, present in fish), and omega-6 (linoleic acid) present in nuts and seeds, particularly as a replacement for saturated fats, have demonstrated beneficial effects on health and a reduction in disease risk and in the case of asthma exerting benefits mainly related with the development and resolution of airway inflammation [41]. Furthermore, the saturated fats, which are highly consumed as part of the Western diet, have pro-inflammatory abilities involved in asthma, amongst other detrimental effects on health. Moreover, the weight loss usually associated to dietary saturated fats' restriction, and the subsequent reduction of adipose tissue, also contributes to a reduction of neutrophilic airway inflammation. This has been recently described in the postprandial period after the intake of foods rich in saturated fatty acids, and also describing that dietary fat is more pro-inflammatory than simple carbohydrates in the case of asthma [42].

It has been reported that individual macronutrients exert a different impact on adipose tissue and inflammatory response [34,43] so that simple sugars and saturated fats, individually and/or combined in the diet, have the ability to induce cytotoxicity and oxidative stress, favoring inflammatory processes and even epigenetically reprogramming the immune response to more severe diseases, as occurs when the Western diet is regularly consumed [44]. Evidences on the negative effect of an unhealthy diet on respiratory health are robust, with dietary components of this type of diet being suggested as pro-inflammatory, inducing to low-grade systemic inflammation and influencing asthma development and severity. Regarding this, studies on the use of the Dietary Inflammatory Index (DII) [45] to predict the anti-inflammatory capacity of the whole diet in the case of asthma are still scarce and warrant further investigation but, they indicate that DII is higher in subjects with asthma and also indicate worse clinical asthma outcomes, indicating that an improvement in this index as an indicator of an adequate diet might be a useful strategy for improving clinical outcomes in asthma [45].

2.2. Role of Food Groups and Dietary Patterns

In this context, the Mediterranean diet reflects a complex concept which includes specific dietary patterns of a high consumption of olive oil as the main source of dietary fats, fruits, green vegetables, nuts, whole cereals, lean protein such as fish, moderate consumption of fermented dairy products and a limited use of meat, meat products and refined sugars [46]. This dietary pattern also includes high consumption of different compounds such as flavonoids, resveratrol or turmeric, among others [43], which are mainly present in vegetables, fruits, olive oil and nuts, and are very powerful against oxidative and inflammatory processes that are highly connected to pathways of the immune system. It is well known that a stable inclusion of this kind of diet, including a wide variety of foods, predominately of plant origin, provides solid health benefits in the prevention and also therapeutic approach of cardiovascular diseases, obesity, type 2 diabetes, metabolic syndrome, cancer and neurodegenerative diseases [47]. Antioxidant and anti-inflammatory properties of compounds present in foods consumed as part of the Mediterranean diet have also demonstrated effectiveness against inflammatory processes and it must be considered that moving away from these dietary patterns usually involves a high intake of processed foods rich in refined starches, sugar and saturated fatty acids that is often accompanied by a lower intake of fish, vegetables, fruits, nuts, legumes and whole grains. Antioxidants are molecules that scavenge free radicals, preventing oxidative damage. If the antioxidant defense system of lungs is unbalanced by oxidants, it can result in pulmonary dysfunction that could be buffered by dietary antioxidants present at high values in plant foods (vitamins C and E, carotene, flavonoids, selenium, etc.). These compounds have been shown to confer a protective effect on neutrophil membranes against oxidants exposure, improving immune cell function and contributing to the positive effect of plant foods' consumption on asthma [48].

However, in the case of the Western diet, it is usually linked to a high consumption of processed foods and also supposes a high presence of saturated fatty acids in addition to a high intake of fat. This kind of dietary fat is strongly linked to inflammation in the adult stage. However, during infancy and childhood, high consumption of these saturated fats may also cause an activation of the innate immune system by excessive production of pro-inflammatory cytokines associated with a reduced production of anti-inflammatory cytokines [49]. This situation must be taken seriously because a gradual shift away from traditional diets to those higher in saturated fats, refined carbohydrates and animal-sourced foods, with increased processed food consumption and also changing culinary practices, has been confirmed [50]. Regarding this, the World Health Organization (WHO) [51] has established a global strategy on diet and health with the aim of reducing unhealthy diets and preventing different diseases, mainly those related to overweight and obesity, including asthma. This improvement of diets includes focusing on promoting fruits, vegetables, legumes, whole grains and nuts, and limiting saturated fats in favor of unsaturated fats, as well as promoting the consumption of foods rich in micronutrients that could reduce associated diseases and mortality.

Processed meats and red meats are also included in the Western dietary pattern and, interestingly, there are studies indicating that a high consumption of these meats has been positively associated with obesity [52]. Regarding this, despite the fact that consumption of cured meats, known for its high nitrite content, may favor airway inflammation and lung damage by nitrosative stress, few studies have been conducted on the association between processed meat and asthma. However, in the case of cured meats, that are an important component of the Western diet, a high intake of this kind of processed meat has been associated with worsening asthma symptoms, probably non-mediated by BMI [53,54], but is important to consider that this Westernized diet includes the consumption of complex meals that might interact with each other and that previous studies [55] have suggested that cured meat may adversely affect lung health, but the magnitude of the cured meat–asthma association may depend on other factors, including obesity or smoking, and must be considered within a broader context, also including dietary patterns and not only cured meat intake. Dietary patterns included in the Mediterranean diet involve a high consumption of fruits and vegetables containing antioxidant compounds that are capable of reducing nitrite levels with an anti-inflammatory effect in lung epithelial cells [55] and probably dampening the effects of high cured meat consumption on asthma symptoms. Moreover, epidemiological studies indicate an increased risk of inflammatory processes when a Mediterranean-style eating pattern is taken away, associated with a high consumption of processed meat, dietary saturated fats and low levels of vitamin D, that can reduce a tolerogenic mucosal immune state locally at the gut but also systemically, and particularly in the lung. In the case of vitamin D, that can be obtained from the diet or by dermal synthesis, its deficiency has been associated with a greater disease activity and extended disease duration in patients with different inflammatory processes, including protection against infections and regulatory effect on the gut microbiota, and has also been linked to beneficial effects in asthma [56].

3. Obesity-Related Asthma and Interrelations with Diet, Inflammation and Adipose Tissue

The parallel trend between the obesity epidemic and asthma makes it necessary to understand mechanisms involved in this association and how different components of foods included in the Western diet can be involved in the regulation of mechanisms in obesity-related asthma. In this regard, there are contradictory studies indicating that obese asthma is poorly controlled by conventional therapies, including corticosteroids, and it shows an increase in neutrophilic airway inflammation; however, there is a growing consensus on the important implication of fatty acids, inducing modifications on lipid metabolism and its immune regulators in obesity-related asthma [57,58]. Obesity has been linked to increased systemic leukotriene inflammation in patients with asthma and the excess of adipose tissue might contribute to airway inflammation, exacerbating asthma symptoms [59]. The inflammatory effect of obese asthma appears to occur through innate immune pathways, with a significant increase in the proportion of neutrophils in the airways of obese asthmatics [57]. In obese asthma, it is important to highlight that body composition and fat distribution affect systemic inflammation, airway inflammation and lung function, and this can explain important differences found between obese males and females with asthma, suggesting that the worsened lung function known to be associated with the obese-asthma phenotype is multifactorial and involves the body composition [60]. Western diet it is usually linked to a high consumption of foods containing important amounts of calories, mainly provided by fats and carbohydrates. In the case of fats, processed foods included in this type of diet provide high amounts of saturated fatty acids in addition to a high intake of fat and calories, increasing the risk of overweight and obesity, that contribute to immune dysfunction as well as altered airway structure and function [61]. The disturbed lipid metabolism and immune modulators of lipid metabolism in obesity, in addition to several immune factors, potentially contributing to the pathogenesis of obesity-related asthma, including intestinal microbiota and inflammation, could indicate that controlled modifications in the diet, in addition to a medical intervention, could be a promising strategy in controlling obesity-related asthma. These modifications in diet (mainly on fats and fiber types and contents) can also exert an important impact on human gut and its microbiome, leading to the selection of a high variety of bacteria interacting both for defense and nutritional advantages. Gut dysbacteriosis might result in altered immune response and chronic inflammatory respiratory disorders, particularly asthma (gut-lung axis), with an important role of the microbiome in inflammation and its influence on important risk factors for asthma being reported. Due to its high content in saturated fats and low fiber content, the Westernized diet can be a major contributor that can trigger factors regulating the development and/or progression of inflammatory conditions, including asthma. Increasing evidence indicates that there is a link between the gut and airways in disease development, reinforcing the evidence on the impact of the Western diet and associated nutrients on immune response and microbiota diversity, and how these can influence the pathology of asthma. Differences found on the lung microbiome between asthmatic and healthy people suggest that bacteria can contribute to the development of asthma, also indicating a possible important role in influencing the immune responses for gut microbiota [62].

Chronic inflammatory diseases are now considered epidemic and highly related with overweight and obesity. All these non-communicable diseases are considered a pandemic of lifestyle-associated pathologies [1]. As findings linking a chronic consumption of Western diet with inflammatory diseases such as asthma are consistent, efforts are now being focused on the study of how diets and combined components of foods can modify immune cell responsiveness. Different microbial metabolites produced after the digestion of foods seem to shed light on how immune cells are shaped in different ways depending on the type of diet. In the case of the Western diet—high in simple sugars and saturated fats—it can alter immune cell responsiveness, inducing systemic inflammation, which plays a key role in asthma patients.

Apart from lipid storage, other biological functions have been attributed to adipose tissue, such as hormones and protein factors' production. These products are known as adipokines, playing different local and systemic roles with the main purpose of the integration of metabolism and immune systems. Pro-inflammatory cytokines such as leptin or resistin are included among them. In the same way, anti-inflammatory adipokines such as adiponectin have also been identified [63–65].

3.1. Anti-Inflammatory Adipokines: Adiponectin

Adiponectin is the best known and most abundant anti-inflammatory adipokine. It is secreted as a monomer, assembling and forming oligomers of different molecular weights. As a result, low, middle and high molecular weight (LMW, MMW and HMW) isoforms have been identified in serum [66] and their receptors, T-cadherin, adipoR1 and adipoR2, are widely distributed. The interaction between adiponectin and Adiponectin receptor 1 (AdipoR) receptors increases intracellular Adenosine monophosphate (AMP) concentration via AMP-activated protein kinase (AMPK) in different tissues and immune cells, with anti-inflammatory effects and AdipoR activation by HMW isoform, and seems capable of reducing tumor necrosis factor-alpha (TNF-α), transforming growth factor beta (TGF-β), interleukin-6 (IL-6) and interleukin-8 (IL-8) cytokines [67]. Adiponectin plasmatic concentration has been mainly associated with adipose tissue repletion, in the way that low calorie intake increases, whereas obesity decreases adiponectin levels [68–70].

Different studies have analyzed the relationship between serum levels of adiponectin and metabolic diseases. In this regard, Zhu et al. [69] and Iwata et al. [70] reported that a high HMW/total adiponectin ratio is positively associated to pheripheric insulin resistance, whereas the association with other isoforms still seems to be unclear. According to the meta-analysis performed by Liu et al. [71], plasmatic levels of adiponectin can be considered as an adequate biomarker for prediction of metabolic syndrome risk. With regard to T-cadherin receptors, they have been related to a protective effect of adiponectin in heart and lung diseases [72]. In fact, different studies based on mice models pointed to the possibility that deficiencies in adiponectin and T-cadherin receptor could be related to myocardial ischemia-hypertrophy and high blood pressure [73–75].

At the bronchio-alveolar epithelium, T-cadherin seems to act as a binding protein, translocating adiponectin from serum to epithelial cells through the capillary barrier, playing an important role in inflammatory response regulation [74,76]. However, this mechanism still remains unclear. On the one hand, Otero et al. [77] proposed that adiponectin could have a pro-inflammatory effect, stimulating epithelial IL-8 secretion. Regarding this, Jaswal et al. [76] recently conducted a cross-sectional observational study comparing adiponectin levels between a group of 60 patients with chronic obstructive pulmonary disease, and 30 healthy people. That study concluded that a high level of adiponectin could have a pro-inflammatory effect, being positively correlated with airway inflammation and inflammatory biomarkers such as IL-8, whereas it was inversely correlated with forced expiratory volume and pulmonary function. On the other hand, Kirdar et al. [78] reported that the presence of a high level of adiponectin could be an attempt to reduce pro-inflammatory cytokines in chronic obstructive pulmonary disease, leading to a downregulation of TNF-α production by macrophages at the bronchio-alveolar epithelium. With regard to asthma, there are no conclusive results about the role of adiponectin on airway inflammation regulation in humans. It seems that serum adiponectin levels would be related to asthma severity, especially in children [79]. Ma et al. [80] analyzed serum adiponectin levels and BMI in 122 asthmatic children, concluding that asthma severity was negatively correlated with adiponectin levels, and positively correlated with BMI. These results are in concordance with previous studies showing that obese and asthmatic children presented an inadequate asthma control and lower serum levels of adiponectin when compared with non-obese asthmatic children [81,82]. The effect of low levels of adiponectin in obese-related asthma could be associated to an increase in TNF-α secretion by macrophages, favoring a Th2-predominant reaction and an eosinophilic-mediated inflammation (type I hyper-sensitivity) [74,82]. Recently, Zhu et al. [83] analyzed the effect of venous adiponectin administration in a murine model of obesity-related asthma, at a cellular and molecular level. According to the results they obtained, obese and asthmatic mice show low levels of serum adiponectin, as well as low levels of lung AdipoR1 and AdipoR2 receptors. Venous administration of adiponectin resulted in a reduction of eosinophils and pulmonary inflammation signs through apoptosis promotion of inflammatory cells, mainly mediated by two mechanisms: downregulation of the inhibitory apoptosis gene Bcl-2, and inhibition of TNF-α secretion. In the same way, administration of adiponectin increased activation of AMPK via AdipoR1 receptors, and inhibited nuclear factor kappa-light-chain-enhancer of activated B cells (NF-kB). Both the activation of AMPK and the inhibition of NF-kB were related to a significant reduction in nitric oxide (NO) species and inducible NO synthase (iNOS), as well as to a significant increment in total antioxidant capacity reported in serum and lung tissue from obese and asthmatic mice.

3.2. Pro-Inflammatory Adipokines: Leptin and Resistin

Leptin was the first adipokine described, being originally defined as a satiety hormone due to its effect on the satiety center in the hypothalamus. Its secretion is mainly regulated by adipocytes' repletion, with its plasmatic levels positively correlating with adipose tissue. When the adipocytes' lipid storage increases, leptin is released in order to stimulate anorexigenic peptides secretion by the hypothalamus [84,85]. However, a pro-inflammatory and immuno-modulatory effect has also been proposed [86,87]. Leptin is a 16 kDa non-glycosylated protein encoded by the *ob*-gene and it is recognized by cell receptors Leptin receptors (LEPRs), which belong to the type I cytokines superfamily. The leptin-LEPR complex activates different intracellular signaling pathways, mainly mediated by four tyrosine Janus Kinases (JAK_1, JAK_2, JAK_3 and tyrosine kinase (TYK_2)) and seven signal transducers and activators of transcription ($STAT_1$–$STAT_7$). Other intracellular pathways activated by leptin are the mitogen-activated protein kinase (MAPK) cascade, the phosphoinositide 3-kinase (PI3K) pathway or the 5′-AMP-activated protein kinase (AMPK) cascade [88]. LEPRs are expressed by the majority of immune cells, where the JAK_2, $STAT_3$, MAPK and PI3K pathways are activated in order to modulate both innate as well as adaptive immune response [44,89]. With regard to innate immune response, leptin promotes cell proliferation and decreases apoptosis, as well as stimulating the activity of NK-cells, activating chemotaxis and the oxidative function of neutrophils, activating the proliferation and pro-inflammatory cytokines release by eosinophils and basophils, or inducing proliferation, activation and pro-inflammatory cytokines production (such as IL-1, IL-2, IL-6, IL-8 or TNF-α) by monocytes, macrophages and dendritic cells. Among leptin's effects on the adaptive immune response, the following have been described: induction of T cell proliferation, polarization to a pro-inflammatory TH_1-IFNγ predominant phenotype instead of to an anti-inflammatory TH_2-IL-4 phenotype, reduction of regulatory T cells and an increment of TH_{17} population favoring the maintenance of inflammatory and auto-immune response, proliferation and activation of B cells' population [90].

Resistin is another adipocyte signaling molecule synthesized not only by adipose tissue, but also by monocytes and macrophages. Its secretion is induced by high glucose levels and inflammatory mediators (lipopolysaccharides, IL-6 or TNFα) [91]. Resistin has been mainly associated to insulin resistance in mice; however, in humans, it seems to actively regulate inflammation. This regulatory effect is mediated by adenylyl cyclase-associated protein-1 (CAP-1) receptors, presented in monocytes and macrophages. Resistin-CAP-1 complex increases intracellular AMP concentration and protein kinase A (PKA) activity, as well as activating DNA transcription regulated by nuclear transcription factor NF-kB. In this way, resistin upregulates the production of pro-inflammatory cytokines such as IL-6, IL-12 or TNFα [90,91].

Based on the above, leptin and resistin have been related to metabolic syndrome- and chronic inflammation-associated diseases. In this way, elevated circulating adipokines levels seem to be involved in the regulation of inflammation and allergic response, affecting the risk of asthma, especially in the case of obesity when adipose tissue is expanded and altered.

As previously explained, obesity has been associated to an increased risk of obstructive airway diseases and severe forms of asthma. In the same way, leptin serum levels are related to obesity and adipocytes' repletion. For these reasons, different studies have tried to elucidate the possible role of leptin in airway inflammation and asthma. Regarding this, Sood et al. [92] performed a cross-sectional study which included 5876 participants (>20 years old), in order to measure basal morning serum levels of leptin, and to establish a possible correlation with clinical asthma status. The results obtained showed that high serum levels of leptin were associated with asthma, and that the association was stronger in women than in men. However, the relationship between BMI, leptin levels and asthma was not corroborated referring to the possible intervention of other factors. In the case of children, Guler et al. [93] also found a positive relationship between asthma and leptin serum levels. Bodini et al. [94] measured the level of leptin in serum and exhaled breath condensate (EBC) in 61 asthmatic and non-asthmatic children from 6 to 14 years old. Those authors also considered the obese and non-obese status based on the BMI. According to the obtained results, although no significant differences were found between obese and obese asthmatic children, they presented significantly higher levels of leptin in EBC and serum than non-obese asthmatic and non-asthmatic children. In the same way, leptin in EBC was significantly higher in non-obese asthmatic children than in non-obese and non-asthmatic children, without differences in serum levels of leptin. From this study, it can be deduced that leptin is able to translocate from serum to the respiratory epithelium, where it could play a crucial role in airway inflammation. This role seems to be more noticeable in non-obese asthmatic children as the systemic pro-inflammatory status and high level of serum leptin in obese children could mask the local airway inflammation.

Less is known about leptin-mediated molecular mechanisms in human airway inflammation and asthma. However, in recent years, different studies conducted on human bronchial cells [95,96] or mice models of obese asthma [97] have shed some light on this mechanism. Hao et al. [95] and Watanabe et al. [96] analyzed the effect of leptin on human bronchial epithelial cells' cultures (HBE16) and human lung fibroblasts, respectively (NHLFs). According to those studies, when HBE16 cells line are exposed to IL-13, mucus secretion would be increased by the upregulation of MUC5AC encoding gene transcription, with this process being mediated by leptin. This mechanism seems to be modulated by leptin activation of the JAK_2-$STAT_3$ intracellular signaling pathway. In parallel, when Normal Human Lung Fibroblasts (NHLFs) cells are cultured under high concentrations of leptin, the production of inflammatory cytokines and myofibroblast differentiation and proliferation is enhanced by the interaction of leptin with LEPR, which is widely expressed by fibroblasts. According to the reported studies, NHLFs stimulation resulted in an induction of chemo-attractants production, including eotaxin, IL-8 or monocyte chemoattractant protein-1 (MCP-1). These cytokines would recruit inflammatory cells, induce cells' degranulation and myofibroblasts differentiation, contributing to asthma exacerbation and epithelial remodeling. With regard to animal models, Chong et al. [97] designed a mice model of obese asthma and after sensitization with intra-parenteral ovalbumin, the animals were sacrificed and bronchoalveolar lavage fluid was collected in order to analyze leptin levels and expression of cellular transcriptional and translational factors. According to their results, leptin levels were higher in Bronchoalveolar lavage (BALF) from obese and asthma-induced animals when compared with non-obese asthmatic and non-asthmatic mice. What is more, when the role of leptin on pulmonary inflammation was analyzed, it was associated to JAK/$STAT_3$ upregulation. As can be seen, studies based on cell cultures and mice models are in concordance, constituting a possible explanation for the mechanism involved in airway inflammation and asthma in humans.

Although the role of resistin in asthma pathogenesis is less known, it has been proposed that resistin serum levels and the resistin:adiponectin ratio could be a predictor of asthma risk and lung function in asthma. Ballantyne et al. [98] conducted a cross-sectional observational study, including 96 asthmatic adults and 46 healthy controls. According to their results, plasmatic resistin levels and the resistin:adiponectin ratio were higher in asthmatic patients than in controls, presenting an inverse correlation with respiratory functional parameters: FEV1% and FEV1/FVC (Forced expiratory volume: FEV; Forced vital capacity: FVC). In the case of the resistin:adiponectin ratio, these differences where higher for obese asthmatic patients, as serum adiponectin levels decrease in obese subjects. However, in contrast to adiponectin, resistin levels were not affected by BMI, which agrees with the previously exposed studies, according to which, resistin secretion is mainly induced by high glucose levels and inflammatory mediators [91]. Different studies have analyzed the resistin-mediated mechanisms in obstructive airway diseases, including asthma. In this respect, Fang et al. [99] analyzed the expression of resistin-like molecule β (p bronchial biopsies from allergic patients, and Resistin-like molecule-beta (RELM-β) effect on both human lung fibroblast cell cultures (MRC5)), and mice previously sensitized and exposed against *Aspergillus fumigatus*. Those authors concluded that RELM-β was highly expressed in airway epithelium from asthmatic patients. Its high expression was associated to the increment of TGF-β local production, which seems to promote proliferation of lung fibroblasts and their differentiation to myofibroblasts. This mechanism would increase subepithelial matrix deposition and would contribute to airway fibrosis, which are crucial for obstructive airway diseases' evolution, such as asthma, since it comprises the reversibility of obstruction. In the same way, Kwak et al. [100] demonstrated that, similar to leptin, resistin increases mucin secretion in human airway epithelial cells through the expression of MUC5AC and MUC5B encoding genes. This mechanism seems to be mediated by NF-Kβ. For that reason, the over-presence of resistin in respiratory epithelium and the over-transcription of MUC encoding genes could be associated to severe asthma, as mucus hypersecretion contributes to airway-obstructive diseases' pathogenesis [101].

In summary, both obesity and adipocytes' repletion have been associated with an imbalance in adipokines' serum concentration, increasing pro-inflammatory adipokines such as leptin or resistin, and decreasing anti-inflammatory cytokines such as adiponectin. In recent years, this imbalance has been related to different inflammatory-related chronic diseases, including asthma. In the case of asthma and obstructive pulmonary disease, pro-inflammatory cytokines seem to increase the risk of asthma and its severity. More specifically, according to the bibliography reviewed, leptin and resistin would lead to an induction of airway inflammation and epithelial proliferation and fibrosis through fibroblast differentiation stimulation and pro-inflammatory cytokines secretion. On the contrary, caloric restriction and adipocytes' depletion are associated to high adiponectin levels in serum, which would decrease local airway inflammation and increase local antioxidant capacity. The previously described mechanisms have been summarized in Figure 1.

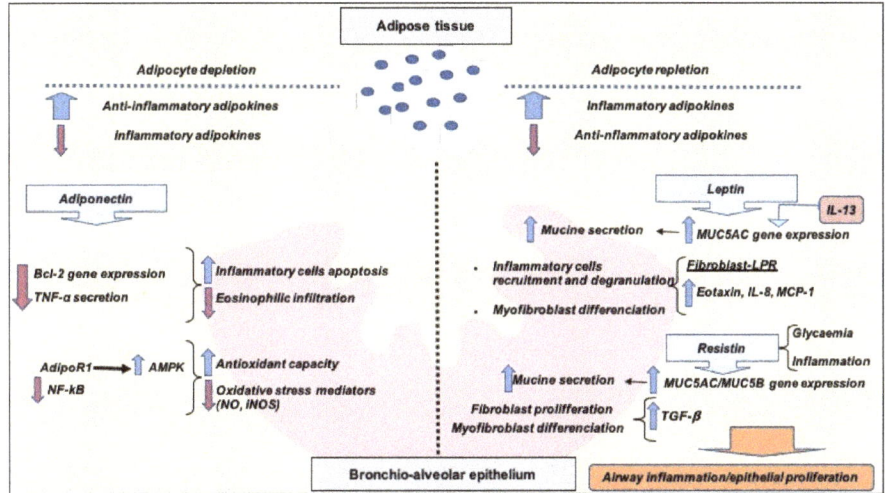

Figure 1. Role of pro-inflammatory and anti-inflammatory adipokines in airway inflammation scheme. Adipocyte depletion is associated with high levels of adiponectin, favoring airway anti-inflammatory status by increasing inflammatory cells' apoptosis and antioxidant capacity, but decreasing eosinophilic infiltration and reducing the production of oxidative stress mediators. This anti-inflammatory status would be mediated by a downregulation of the inhibitory apoptosis gene Bcl-2, inhibition of TNF-α secretion by airway macrophages and the increment of intracellular AMP-kinase activity through activation of AdipoR1 receptors. A pro-inflammatory cytokine such as leptin is related to obesity and adipocytes' repletion, whereas resistin levels are increased under high glycaemia and the influence of inflammatory factors. Both leptin and resistin high levels would increase airway mucin secretion through MUC-gene expression, as well as favoring fibroblast proliferation, myofibroblast differentiation and local inflammatory cells' recruitment through the secretion of pro-inflammatory cytokines (Eotaxin, IL-8, MCP-1 or TGF-β). In this way, high plasmatic levels of leptin and resistin could favor airway inflammation and epithelial remodeling, which are crucial for pulmonary obstructive diseases' severity and their evolution. Abbreviations: TNF, tumor necrosis factor; NO, nitric oxide; iNOS, inducible nitric oxide synthase isoforms; AmpK, AMP-activated protein kinase; Bcl-2, B-cell lymphoma type 2 gene; NF-kB, nuclear factor kappa-light-chain-enhancer of activated cells; IL, interleukin; MUC5AC Mucin 5AC precursor gene; TGF-β, Tumor growth factor b; MCP-1, Monocyte chemoattractant protein-1.

4. Concluding Remarks and Future Directions

Dietary patterns play a main role in the risk and development of many diseases, including asthma. Western lifestyle implies a regular intake of foods containing high amounts of saturated fats and simple sugars that also suppose a reduced intake of complex carbohydrates, unsaturated fats and antioxidant compounds present in plant-origin food. In this frame, the obesity epidemic is highly related with Western/unhealthy dietary patterns and with the alarming and simultaneous growth of inflammatory diseases such as asthma. Related to this, more information about the risk associated with Westernized lifestyles should be managed in order to avoid a detrimental reprogramming of the immune response to be more inflammatory, which can lead to more severe diseases, as occurs when a Western diet is regularly consumed. Dietary management, encouraging the consumption of unsaturated fats rather than foods rich in saturated fats, and promoting the consumption of whole grain-derived foods and plant-origin foods, will provide a diet with anti-inflammatory properties and, probably, with a positive effect on adipose tissue and airway inflammatory processes. Thus, incorporating adequate dietary patterns promoting the Mediterranean diet and insisting on the importance of reducing the intake of sugar-sweetened beverages and highly processed foods into the clinical management of asthma is to be highly recommended.

Author Contributions: L.G.-M. had the original idea for this manuscript.; C.F.-S., C.A.G.-B. and L.G.-M. wrote the paper. All authors approved the final version of the manuscript.

Funding: This research received no external funding.

Conflicts of Interest: The authors confirm that this article content has no conflict of interest.

References

1. Christ, A.; Latz, E. The Western lifestyle has lasting effects on metaflammation. *Nat. Rev. Immunol.* **2019**, *19*, 267–268. [CrossRef]
2. Periyalil, H.A.; Wood, L.G.; Wright, T.A.; Karihaloo, C.; Starkey, M.R.; Miu, A.S.; Baines, K.J.; Hansbro, P.M.; Gibson, P.G. Obese asthmatics are characterized by altered adipose tissue macrophage activation. *Clin. Exp. Allergy* **2018**, *48*, 641–649. [CrossRef] [PubMed]
3. Sin, D.D.; Sutherland, E.R. Obesity and the lung: 4. Obesity and asthma. *Thorax* **2008**, *63*, 1018–1023. [CrossRef] [PubMed]
4. Rush, E.C.; Yan, M.R. Evolution not Revolution: Nutrition and Obesity. *Nutrients* **2017**, *9*, 519. [CrossRef] [PubMed]
5. Braback, L.; Hjern, A.; Rasmussen, F. Trends in asthma, allergic rhinitis and eczema among Swedish conscripts from farming and non-farming environments. A nationwide study over three decades. *Clin. Exp. Allergy* **2004**, *34*, 38–43. [CrossRef]
6. Haahtela, T.; Lindholm, H.; Bjorksten, F.; Koskenvuo, K.; Laitinen, L.A. Prevalence of asthma in Finnish young men. *BMJ* **1990**, *301*, 266–268. [CrossRef]
7. Eder, W.; Ege, M.J.; von Mutius, E. The asthma epidemic. *N. Engl. J. Med.* **2006**, *355*, 2226–2235. [CrossRef]
8. García-Marcos, L.; Quiros, A.B.; Hernández, G.G.; Guillen-Grima, F.; Díaz, C.G.; Ureña, I.C.; Peña, A.A.; Monge, R.B.; Suarez-Varela, M.M.; Varela, A.L.; et al. Stabilization of asthma prevalence among adolescents and increase among schoolchildren (ISAAC phases I and III) in Spain. *Allergy* **2004**, *59*, 1301–1307. [CrossRef]
9. Asher, M.I.; Montefort, S.; Bjorksten, B.; Lai, C.K.; Strachan, D.P.; Weiland, S.K.; Williams, H. Worldwide time trends in the prevalence of symptoms of asthma, allergic rhinoconjunctivitis, and eczema in childhood: ISAAC Phases One and Three repeat multicountry cross-sectional surveys. *Lancet* **2006**, *368*, 733–743. [CrossRef]
10. Hales, C.M.; Fryar, C.D.; Carroll, M.D.; Freedman, D.S.; Ogden, C.L. Trends in Obesity and Severe Obesity Prevalence in US Youth and Adults by Sex and Age, 2007–2008 to 2015–2016. *JAMA* **2018**, *319*, 1723–1725. [CrossRef]
11. Ogden, C.L.; Fryar, C.D.; Hales, C.M.; Carroll, M.D.; Aoki, Y.; Freedman, D.S. Differences in Obesity Prevalence by Demographics and Urbanization in US Children and Adolescents, 2013–2016. *JAMA* **2018**, *319*, 2410–2418. [CrossRef] [PubMed]
12. Hallstrand, T.S.; Fischer, M.E.; Wurfel, M.M.; Afari, N.; Buchwald, D.; Goldberg, J. Genetic pleiotropy between asthma and obesity in a community-based sample of twins. *J. Allergy Clin. Immunol.* **2005**, *116*, 1235–1241. [CrossRef] [PubMed]
13. Thomsen, S.F.; Ulrik, C.S.; Kyvik, K.O.; Sørensen, T.I.; Posthyma, D.; Skadhauge, L.R.; Steffensen, I.; Backer, V. Association between obesity and asthma in a twin cohort. *Allergy* **2007**, *62*, 1199–1204. [CrossRef] [PubMed]
14. Garcia-Marcos, L.; Canflanca, I.M.; Garrido, J.B.; Varela, A.L.; Garcia-Hernandez, G.; Guillen-Grima, F.; Gonzalez-Diaz, C.; Carbajal-Ureña, I.; Arnedo-Peña, A.; Busquets-Monge, R.M.; et al. Relationship of asthma and rhinoconjunctivitis with obesity, exercise and Mediterranean diet in Spanish schoolchildren. *Thorax* **2007**, *62*, 503–508. [CrossRef] [PubMed]
15. Garcia-Marcos, L.; Castro-Rodriguez, J.A.; Weinmayer, G.; Panagiotakos, D.B.; Priftis, K.N.; Nagel, G. Influence of Mediterranean diet on asthma in children: A systematic review and meta-analysis. *Pediatr. Allergy Immunol.* **2013**, *24*, 330–338. [CrossRef] [PubMed]
16. Ellwood, P.; Asher, M.I.; Garcia-Marcos, L.; Williams, H.; Keil, U.; Robertson, C.; Nagel, G. Do fast foods cause asthma, rhinoconjunctivitis and eczema? Global findings from the International Study of Asthma and Allergies in Childhood (ISAAC) phase three. *Thorax* **2013**, *68*, 351–360. [CrossRef]

17. Papadopoulou, A.; Panagiotakos, D.B.; Hatziagorou, E.; Antonogeorgos, G.; Matziou, V.N.; Tsanakas, J.N.; Gratziou, C.; Tsabouri, S.; Priftis, K.N. Antioxidant foods consumption and childhood asthma and other allergic diseases: The Greek cohorts of the ISAAC II survey. *Allergol. Immunopathol. (Madr)* **2015**, *43*, 353–360. [CrossRef]
18. Sahiner, U.M.; Birben, E.; Erzurum, S.; Sackesen, C.; Kalayci, O. Oxidative stress in asthma: Part of the puzzle. *Pediatr. Allergy Immunol.* **2018**, *29*, 789–800. [CrossRef]
19. Wall, C.R.; Stewart, A.W.; Hancox, R.J.; Murphy, R.; Braithwaite, I.; Beasley, R.; Mitchell, E.A. Association between frequency counsumption of fruit, vegetables, nuts and pulses and BMI: Alayses of the International study of Asthma and Allergies in Childhood. *Nutrients* **2018**, *10*, 316. [CrossRef]
20. Amati, F.; Hassounah, S.; Swaka, A. The Impact of Mediterranean Dietary Patterns During Pregnancy on Maternal and Offspring Health. *Nutrients* **2019**, *11*, 1098. [CrossRef]
21. Forno, E.; Young, O.M.; Kumar, R.; Simhan, H.; Celedon, J.C. Maternal obesity in pregnancy, gestional weight gain and risk of childhood asthma. *Pediatrics* **2014**, *134*, e535–e546. [CrossRef] [PubMed]
22. Tie, H.T.; Xia, Y.Y.; Zeng, Y.S.; Zhang, Y.; Dai, C.L.; Guo, J.J.; Zhao, Y. Risk of childhood overweight or obesity associated with excessive weight gain during pregnancy: A meta-analysis. *Arch. Gynecol. Obstet.* **2014**, *289*, 247–257. [CrossRef]
23. Nagel, G.; Weinmayr, G.; Kleiner, A.; García-Marcos, L.; Strachan, D.P. Effect of diet on asthma and allergic sensitization in the International Studies on Allergies and Asthma in Childhood (ISAAC) Phase Two. *Thorax* **2010**, *65*, 516–522. [CrossRef] [PubMed]
24. Alwarith, J.; Kahleova, H.; Crosby, L.; Brooks, A.; Brandon, L.; Levin, S.M.; Barnard, N.D. The role of nutrition in asthma prevention and treatment. *Nutr. Rev.* **2020**. [CrossRef] [PubMed]
25. Schulze, M.B.; Martínez-González, M.A.; Fung, T.T.; Lichtenstein, A.H.; Forouhi, N.H. Food based dietary patterns and chronic disease prevention. *BMJ* **2018**, *361*, k2396. [CrossRef] [PubMed]
26. Younas, H.; Vieira, M.; Gu, C.; Lee, R.; Shin, M.K.; Berger, S.; Loube, J.; Nelson, A.; Bevans-Fonti, S.; Zhong, Q.; et al. Caloric restriction prevents the development of airway hyperresponsiveness in mice on a high fat diet. *Sci. Rep.* **2019**, *22*, 279. [CrossRef]
27. Castro Rodríguez, J.A.; Garcia Marcos, L. What is the effect of a Mediterranean diet on allergies and asthma in children? *Front. Pediatr.* **2017**, *21*, 72. [CrossRef]
28. Brandhorst, S.; Longo, V.D. Dietary restrictions and nutrition in the prevention and treatment of cardiovascular disease. *Circ. Res.* **2019**, *124*, 952–965. [CrossRef]
29. López-Guarnido, O.; Urquiza, N.; Saiz, M.; Lozano, D.; Rodrigo, L.; Pascual, M.; Lorente, J.A.; Alvarez-Cubero, M.J.; Rivas, A. Bioactive compounds of the Mediterranean diet and prostate cancer. *Aging Male* **2018**, *21*, 251–260. [CrossRef]
30. Brigham, E.P.; Kolahdooz, F.; Hansel, N.; Breysse, P.N.; Davis, M.; Sharma, S.; Matsui, E.C.; Diette, G.; McCormack, M.C. Association between Western diet pattern and adult asthma: A focused review. *Ann. Allergy Asthma Immunol.* **2015**, *114*, 273–280. [CrossRef]
31. Park, Y.; Subar, A.F.; Hollenbeck, A.; Schatzkin, A. Dietary fiber intake and mortality in the NIH-AARP diet and health study. *Arch. Intern. Med.* **2011**, *171*, 1061–1068. [CrossRef] [PubMed]
32. Calder, P.C. Omega-3 polyunsaturated fatty acids and inflammatory processes: Nutrition or pharmacology? *Br. J. Clin. Pharmacol.* **2013**, *75*, 645–662. [CrossRef] [PubMed]
33. Andersen, C.J.; Fernandez, M.L. Dietary strategies to reduce metabolic syndrome. *Rev. Endocr. Metab. Dis.* **2013**, *14*, 241–254. [CrossRef] [PubMed]
34. Sarin, H.V.; Lee, H.; Jauhiainen, M.; Joensuu, A.; Borodulin, K.; Männistö, S.; Jin, Z.; Terwilliger, J.D.; Isola, V.; Ahtiainen, P.; et al. Substantial fat mass loss reduces low-grade inflammation and induces positive alteration in cardiometabolic factors in normal-weight individuals. *Nat. Sci. Rep.* **2019**, *9*, 3450. [CrossRef] [PubMed]
35. Duwaerts, C.C.; Maher, J.J. Macronutrients and the adipose-liver axis in obesity and fatty liver. *Cell. Mol. Gastroenterol. Hepatol.* **2019**, *7*, 749–761. [CrossRef]
36. Ellulu, M.S.; Patimah, I.; Khazáai, H.; Rahmat, A.; Abed, Y. Obesity and inflammation: The linking mechanism and the complications. *Arch. Med. Sci.* **2017**, *13*, 851–863. [CrossRef]
37. Maggini, S.; Pierre, A.; Calder, P.C. Immune function and micronutrient requirements change over the life course. *Nutrients* **2018**, *10*, 1531. [CrossRef]

38. Jensen, M.K.; Koh-Banerjee, P.; Franz, M.; Sampson, L.; Gronbaek, M.; Rimm, E.B. Whole grains, bran and germ in relation to homocysteine and markers of glycemic control, lipids and inflammation. *Am. J. Clin. Nutr.* **2006**, *83*, 275–283. [CrossRef]
39. Boulangé, C.L.; Neves, A.L.; Chilloux, J.; Nicholson, J.K.; Dumas, M.E. Impact of the gut microbiota, obesity, and metabolic disease. *Genome Med.* **2016**, *8*, 42. [CrossRef]
40. DeChristopher, L.R.; Tucker, K.L. Excess of free fructose, high-fructose corn syrup and adult asthma: The Framingham Offspring Cohort. *Br. J. Nutr.* **2018**, *119*, 1157–1167. [CrossRef]
41. Botchlett, R.; Chaodong, W. Diet composition for the management of obesity and obesity-related disorders. *J. Diabetes Mellit. Metab. Syndr.* **2018**, *3*, 10–25. [CrossRef] [PubMed]
42. Wendel, S.G.; Baffi, C.; Holguin, F. Fatty acids, inflammation and asthma. *J. Allergy Clin. Inmunol.* **2014**, *133*, 1255–1264. [CrossRef]
43. Sureda, A.; Bibiloni, M.M.; Julibert, A.; Bouzas, C.; Argelich, E.; Llompart, I.; Pons, A.; Tur, J.A. Adherence to the Mediterranean Diet and inflammatory markers. *Nutrients* **2018**, *10*, 62. [CrossRef] [PubMed]
44. Wood, L.G.; Li, Q.; Scott, H.A.; Rutting, S.; Berthon, B.S.; Gibson, P.G.; Hansbro, P.M.; Williams, E.; Horvat, J.; Simpson, J.L.; et al. Saturated fatty acids, obesity, and the nucleotide oligomerization domain-like receptor protein 3 (NLRP3) inflammasome in asthmatic patients. *J. Allergy Clin. Inmunol.* **2019**, *143*, 305–315. [CrossRef] [PubMed]
45. Wood, L.G.; Shivappa, N.; Berthon, B.S.; Gibson, P.G.; Hebert, J.R. Dietary inflammatory index is related to asthma risk, lung function and systemic inflammation in asthma. *Clin. Exp. Allergy* **2015**, *45*, 177–183. [CrossRef]
46. Kim, J.H.; Elwood, P.E.; Asher, M.I. Diet and asthma: Looking back, moving forward. *Respir. Res.* **2009**, *10*, 49. [CrossRef]
47. Dandona, P.; Ghanim, H.; Chaudhuri, A.; Dhindsa, S.; Kim, S.S. Macronutrient intake induces oxidative and inflammatory stress: Potential relevance to atherosclerosis and insulin resistance. *Exp. Mol. Med.* **2010**, *42*, 245–253. [CrossRef]
48. Sofi, F.; Macchi, C.; Abbate, R.; Gensini, G.F.; Casini, A. Mediterranean diet and health. *Biofactors* **2013**, *39*, 335–342. [CrossRef]
49. Te Morenga, L.; Montez, J.M. Health effects of saturated and trans-fatty acid intake in children and adolescents: Systematic review and meta-analysis. *PLoS ONE* **2017**, *12*, e0186672. [CrossRef]
50. Sievert, K.; Lawrence, M.; Naika, A.; Baker, P. Processed foods and nutrition transition in the Pacific: Regional trends, patterns and food system drivers. *Nutrients* **2019**, *11*, 1328. [CrossRef]
51. WHO. *Essential Nutrition Actions: Mainstreaming Nutrition throughout the Life-Course*; World Health Organization: Geneva, Switzerland, 2019; ISBN 978-92-4-151585-6.
52. Li, Z.; Rava, M.; Bédard, A.; Dumas, O.; Garcia-Aymerich, J.; Leynaert, B.; Pison, C.; Le Moual, N.; Romieu, I.; Siroux, V.; et al. Cured meat intake is associated with worsening asthma symptoms. *Thorax* **2017**, *72*, 206–212. [CrossRef]
53. Brathwaite, N.; Fraser, H.S.; Modeste, N.; Broome, H.; King, R. Obesity, diabetes, hypertension, and vegetarian status among Seventh-Day Adventists in Barbados: Preliminary results. *Ethn. Dis.* **2003**, *13*, 34–39.
54. Andrianasolo, R.; Kesse-Guyot, E.; Moufidath, A.; Hercberg, S.; Galan, P.; Varraso, R. Association between cured meat intake and asthma symptoms. *Eur. Respir. J.* **2018**, *52*, PA1149.
55. Statovci, D.; Aguilera, M.; MacSharry, J.; Melgar, S. The impact of Western diet and nutrients on the microbiota and immune response at mucosal interfaces. *Front. Immunol.* **2017**, *8*, 38. [CrossRef] [PubMed]
56. Pfeffer, P.E.; Hawrylowicz, C.M. Vitamin D in asthma. Mechanisms of action and considerations for clinical trials. *CHEST* **2018**, *153*, 1229–1239. [CrossRef] [PubMed]
57. Scott, H.A.; Gibson, P.G.; Garg, M.L.; Wood, L.G. Airway inflammation is augmented by obesity and fatty acids in asthma. *Eur. Respir. J.* **2011**, *38*, 594–602. [CrossRef]
58. Umetsu, D.T. Mechanisms by which obesity impacts upon asthma. *Thorax* **2017**, *72*, 174–177. [CrossRef]
59. Pérez-Pérez, A.; Vilariño-García, T.; Fernández-Riejos, P.; Martín-González, J.; Segura-Egea, J.J.; Sánchez-Margalet, V. Role of leptin as a link between metabolism and the immune system. *Cytokine Growth Factor Rev.* **2017**, *35*, 71–84. [CrossRef]
60. Scott, H.A.; Gibson, P.G.; Garg, M.L.; Pretto, J.J.; Morgan, P.J.; Callister, R.; Wood, L.G. Relationship between body composition, inflammation and lung function in overweight and obese asthma. *Respir. Res.* **2012**, *13*, 10. [CrossRef]

61. Dixon, A.A.; Poynter, M.E. Mechanisms of asthma in obesity: Pleiotropic aspects of obesity produce distinct asthma phenotypes. *Am. J. Respir. Cell Mol. Biol.* **2016**, *54*, 601–608. [CrossRef]
62. Frati, F.; Salvatori, C.; Incorvaia, C.; Bellucci, A.; Di Cara, G.; Marcucci, F.; Esposito, S. The role of the microbiome in asthma: The gut-lung axis. *Int. J. Mol. Sci.* **2019**, *20*, 123. [CrossRef] [PubMed]
63. Samir, P.; Malireddi, S.; Kanneganti, T.D. Food for training- Western diet and inflammatory memory. *Cell Metab.* **2018**, *27*, 481–482. [CrossRef] [PubMed]
64. Trayhurn, P.; Wood, I.S. Adipokines: Inflammation and the pleiotropic role of white adipose tissue. *Br. J. Nutr.* **2004**, *92*, 347–355. [CrossRef] [PubMed]
65. Mancuso, P. The role of adipokines in chronic inflammation. *Immunotargets Ther.* **2016**, *5*, 47–56. [CrossRef]
66. Ambroszkiewicz, J.; Chełchowska, M.; Rowicka, G.; Klemarczyk, W.; Strucińska, M.; Gajewska, J. Anti-Inflammatory and Pro-Inflammatory Adipokine Profiles in Children on vegetarian and Omnivorous Diets. *Nutrients* **2018**, *10*, 1241. [CrossRef]
67. Peake, P.W.; Kriketos, A.D.; Campbell, L.V.; Shen, Y.; Charlesworth, J.A. The metabolism of isoforms of human adiponectin: Studies in human subjects and in experimental animals. *Eur. J. Endocrinol.* **2005**, *153*, 409–417. [CrossRef]
68. Salehi-Abargouei, A.; Izadi, V.; Azadbakht, L. The effect of low calorie diet on adiponectin concentration: A systematic review and meta-analysis. *Horm. Metab. Res.* **2015**, *47*, 549–555. [CrossRef]
69. Zhu, N.; Pankow, J.S.; Ballantyne, C.M.; Couper, D.; Hoogeveen, R.C.; Pereira, M.; Duncan, B.B.; Schmidt, M.I. High-molecular-weight adiponectin and the risk of type 2 diabetes in the ARIC study. *J. Clin. Endocrinol. Metab.* **2010**, *95*, 5097–5104. [CrossRef] [PubMed]
70. Iwata, M.; Hara, K.; Kamura, Y.; Honoki, H.; Fujisaka, S.; Ishiki, M.; Usui, I.; Yagi, K.; Fukushima, Y.; Takano, A.; et al. Ratio of low molecular weight serum adiponectin to the total adiponectin value is associated with type 2 diabetes through its relation to increasing insulin resistance. *PLoS ONE* **2018**, *13*, e0192609. [CrossRef] [PubMed]
71. Liu, Z.; Liang, S.; Que, S.; Zhou, L.; Zheng, S.; Mardinoglu, A. Meta-analysis of adiponectin as a biomarker for the detection of metabolic syndrome. *Front. Physiol.* **2018**, *9*, 1–16. [CrossRef] [PubMed]
72. Nigro, E.; Daniele, A.; Scudiero, O.; Ludovica-Monaco, M.; Roviezzo, F.; D'Agostino, B.; Mazzarella, G.; Bianco, A. Adiponectin in asthma: Implications for phenotyping. *Curr. Protein Pept. Sci.* **2015**, *16*, 182–187. [CrossRef] [PubMed]
73. Denzel, M.S.; Scimia, M.C.; Zumstein, P.M.; Walsh, K.; RuizLozano, P.; Ranscht, B. T-cadherin is critical for adiponectin mediated cardioprotection in mice. *J. Clin. Investig.* **2010**, *120*, 4342–4352. [CrossRef] [PubMed]
74. Parker-Duffen, J.L.; Nakamura, K.; Silver, M.; Kikuchi, R.; Tigges, U.; Yoshida, S.; Denzel, M.S.; Ranscht, B.; Walsh, K. T-cadherin is essential for adiponectin-mediated revascularization. *J. Biol. Chem.* **2013**, *288*, 24886–24897. [CrossRef] [PubMed]
75. Kalisz, M.; Baranowska, B.; Wolińska-Witort, E.; Mączewski, M.; Mackiewicz, U.; Tułacz, D.; Gora, M.; Martynska, L.; Bik, W. Total and high molecular weight adiponectin levels in the rat model of post-myocardial infarction heart failure. *J. Physiol. Pharmacol.* **2015**, *66*, 673–680.
76. Jaswal, S.; Saini, V.; Kaur, J.; Gupta, S.; Kaur, H.; Garg, K. Association of Adiponectin with Lung Function Impairment and Disease Severity in Chronic Obstructive Pulmonary Disease. *Int. J. Appl. Basic. Med. Res.* **2018**, *8*, 14–18. [CrossRef] [PubMed]
77. Otero, M.; Lago, R.; Gomez, R.; Lago, F.; Dieguez, C.; Gómez-Reino, J.J.; Gualillo, O. Changes in plasma levels of fat-derived hormones adiponectin, leptin, resistin and visfatin in patients with rheumatoid arthritis. *Ann. Rheum. Dis.* **2006**, *65*, 1198–1201. [CrossRef] [PubMed]
78. Kirdar, S.; Serter, M.; Ceylan, E.; Sener, A.G.; Kavak, T.; Karadağ, F. Adiponectin as a biomarker of systemic inflammatory response in smoker patients with stable and exacerbation phases of chronic obstructive pulmonary disease. *Scand. J. Clin. Lab. Investig.* **2009**, *69*, 219–224. [CrossRef] [PubMed]
79. Sood, A.; Shore, S.A. Adiponectin, leptin, and resistin in asthma: Basic mechanisms through population studies. *J. Allergy* **2013**, *2013*, e785835. [CrossRef]
80. Ma, C.; Wang, Y.; Xue, M. Correlations of severity of asthma in children with body mass index, adiponectin and leptin. *J. Clin. Lab. Anal.* **2019**, *33*, e22915. [CrossRef]
81. Wahab, A.; Maarafiya, M.M.; Ashraf Soliman, A.; Noura, B.M.; Younes, N.B.M.; Chandra, P. Serum Leptin and Adiponectin Levels in Obese and Nonobese Asthmatic School Children in relation to Asthma Control. *J. Allergy* **2013**, *2013*, e654104.

82. Yuksel, H.; Sogut, A.; Yilmaz, O.; Onur, E.; Dinc, G. Role of adipokines and hormones of obesity in childhood asthma. *Allergy Asthma Immunol. Res.* **2012**, *4*, 98–103. [CrossRef] [PubMed]
83. Zhu, L.; Chen, X.; Chong, L.; Kong, L.; Wen, S.; Zhang, H.; Zhang, W.; Li, C. Adiponectin alleviates exacerbation of airway inflammation and oxidative stress in obesity-related asthma mice partly through AMPK signaling pathway. *Int. Immunopharmacol.* **2019**, *67*, 396–407. [CrossRef] [PubMed]
84. Friedman, J.M.; Halaas, J.L. Leptin and the regulation of body weight in mammals. *Nature* **1998**, *395*, 763–770. [CrossRef] [PubMed]
85. Heisler, L.K.; Lam, D.D. An appetite for life: Brain regulation of hunger and satiety. *Curr. Opin. Pharmacol.* **2017**, *37*, 100–106. [CrossRef]
86. Otero, M.; Lago, R.; Gomez, R.; Dieguez, C.; Lago, F.; Gomez-Reino, J.; Gualillo, O. Towards a pro-inflammatory and immunomodulatory emerging role of leptin. *Rheumatology* **2006**, *45*, 944–950. [CrossRef]
87. Frühbeck, G. Intracellular signalling pathways activated by leptin. *Biochem. J.* **2006**, *393*, 7–20. [CrossRef]
88. Abella, V.; Scotece, M.; Conde, J.; Pino, J.; Gonzalez-Gay, M.A.; Gomez-Reino, J.J.; Mera, A.; Lago, F.; Gomez, R.; Gualillo, O. Leptin in the interplay of inflammation, metabolism and immune system disorders. *Nat. Rev. Rheumatol.* **2017**, *13*, 100–109. [CrossRef] [PubMed]
89. Schwartz, D.R.; Lazar, M.A. Human resistin: Found in translation from mouse to man. *Trends Endocrinol. Metab.* **2011**, *22*, 259–265. [CrossRef] [PubMed]
90. Lee, S.; Lee, H.C.; Kwon, Y.W.; Lee, S.E.; Cho, Y.; Kim, J.; Lee, S.; Kim, J.Y.; Lee, J.; Yang, H.M.; et al. Adenylyl cyclase-associated protein 1 is a receptor for human resistin and mediates inflammatory actions of human monocytes. *Cell Metab.* **2014**, *4*, 484–497. [CrossRef] [PubMed]
91. Park, H.K.; Kwak, M.K.; Kim, H.J.; Ahima, R.S. Linking resistin, inflammation, and cardiometabolic diseases. *Korean J. Intern. Med.* **2017**, *32*, 239–247. [CrossRef]
92. Sood, A.; Ford, E.S.; Camargo, C.A. Association between leptin and asthma in adults. *Thorax* **2006**, *61*, 300–305. [CrossRef]
93. Guler, N.; Kirerleri, E.; Ones, U.; Tamay, Z.; Salmayenli, N.; Darendeliler, F. Leptin: Does it have any role in childhood asthma? *J. Allergy Clin. Immunol.* **2004**, *114*, 254–259. [CrossRef] [PubMed]
94. Bodini, A.; Tenero, L.; Sandri, M.; Maffeis, C.; Piazza, M.; Zanoni, L.; Peroni, D.; Boner, A.; Piacentini, G. Serum and exhaled breath condensate leptin levels in asthmatic and obesity children: A pilot study. *J. Breath Res.* **2017**, *11*, 046005. [CrossRef] [PubMed]
95. Hao, W.; Wang, J.; Zhang, Y.; Wang, Y.; Sun, L.; Han, W. Leptin positively regulates MUC5AC production and secretion induced by interleukin-13 in human bronchial epithelial cells. Biochem Biophys. *Res. Commun.* **2017**, *493*, 979–984.
96. Watanabe, K.; Suzukawa, M.; Arakawa, S.; Kobayashi, K.; Igarashi, S.; Tashimo, H.; Nagai, H.; Tohma, S.; Nagase, T.; Ohta, K. Leptin enhances cytokine/chemokine production by normal lung fibroblasts by binding to leptin receptor. *Allergol. Int.* **2019**, *68*, S3–S8. [CrossRef]
97. Chong, L.; Liu, L.; Zhu, L.; Li, H.; Shao, Y.; Zhang, H.; Yu, G. Expression Levels of Predominant Adipokines and Activations of STAT3, STAT6 in an Experimental Mice Model of Obese Asthma. *Iran. J. Allergy Asthma Immunol.* **2019**, *18*, 62–71. [CrossRef] [PubMed]
98. Ballantyne, D.; Scott, H.; MacDonald-Wicks, L.; Gibson, P.G.; Wood, L.G. Resistin is a predictor of asthma risk and resistin: Adiponectin ratio is a negative predictor of lung function in asthma. *Clin. Exp. Allergy* **2016**, *46*, 1056–1065. [CrossRef] [PubMed]
99. Fang, C.L.; Yin, L.J.; Sharma, S.; Kierstein, S.; Wu, H.F.; Eid, G.; Haczku, A.; Corrigan, C.J.; Ying, S. Resistin-like molecule-β (RELM-β) targets airways fibroblasts to effect remodelling in asthma: From mouse to man. *Clin. Exp. Allergy* **2015**, *45*, 940–952. [CrossRef]
100. Kwak, S.; Kim, Y.D.; Na, H.G.; Bae, C.H.; Song, S.Y.; Choi, Y.S. Resistin upregulates MUC5AC/B mucin gene expression in human airway epithelial cells. *Biochem. Biophys. Res. Commun.* **2018**, *499*, 655–661. [CrossRef]
101. Lachowicz-Scroggins, M.E.; Yuan, S.; Kerr, S.C.; Dunican, E.M.; Yu, M.; Carrington, S.D.; Fahy, J.V. Abnormalities in MUC5AC and MUC5B protein in airway mucus in asthma. *Am. J. Respir. Crit. Care Med.* **2016**, *194*, 1296–1299. [CrossRef]

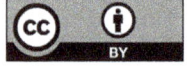

© 2020 by the authors. Licensee MDPI, Basel, Switzerland. This article is an open access article distributed under the terms and conditions of the Creative Commons Attribution (CC BY) license (http://creativecommons.org/licenses/by/4.0/).

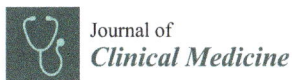

Article

Preschool Asthma Symptoms in Children Born Preterm: The Relevance of Lung Function in Infancy

Manuel Sanchez-Solis [1,2,3,*], Maria Soledad Parra-Carrillo [2], Pedro Mondejar-Lopez [1,2], Patricia W Garcia-Marcos [1] and Luis Garcia-Marcos [1,2,3]

1. Pediatric Pulmonology Unit, Virgen de la Arrixaca University Hospital, Murcia University, 30003 Murcia, Spain; mondejarp@gmail.com (P.M.-L.); part.garcia.marcos@gmail.com (P.W.G.-M.); lgmarcos@um.es (L.G.-M.)
2. Department of Surgery, Pediatrics, Obstetrics and Gynecology, University of Murcia, 30003 Murcia, Spain; mariasoledadparrac@gmail.com
3. Arrixaca Bioresearch Institute of Murcia, 30003 Murcia, Spain
* Correspondence: msolis@um.es; Tel.: +34-968-369-606

Received: 30 July 2020; Accepted: 7 October 2020; Published: 18 October 2020

Abstract: Background: The aim of the study is to assess whether lung function of infants born preterm predicts wheezing in pre-school age. **Methods:** A survey of the core wheezing questionnaire of the International Study on Asthma and Allergy in Children was administered to parents of preterm newborns, to whom lung function tests were performed at a corrected age of six months, and who, at the time of the survey, were between three and nine years of age. **Results:** Low values of all lung function parameters measured, except FVC, were predictors of wheezing at some time in life, (FEV0.5 OR: 0.62 (95%CI 0.39; 0.995); FEV0.5/FVC OR: 0.73 (0.54; 0.99)) FEF75 OR: 0.60 [0.37; 0.93]; FEF25-75 OR: 0.57 (0.37; 0.89)); and of wheezing in the past year (FEV0.5 OR: 0.36 (0.17; 0.76); FEV0.5/FVC OR: 0.59 (0.38; 0.93); FEF75 OR: 0.38 [0.19; 0.76]; FEF25-75 OR: 0.35 (0.17; 0.70). In addition, FEV0.5/FVC values lower than the lowest limit of normality, were predictive of hospital admissions due to wheezing (OR: 3.07; (1.02; 9.25)). **Conclusions:** Limited lung function in infancy is predictive of both future wheezing and hospitalization for a wheezing episode.

Keywords: pre-school asthma; preterm newborn; infant lung function

1. Introduction

According to previous studies, children born preterm have an increased risk of wheeze and asthma as compared to children born at term. This risk is higher when gestational age is lower [1] and is independent of a family history of atopy [2]. Additionally, preterm children have lower lung function during their infancy than their counterparts born at term [3,4] and this low lung function persists until school age [5,6] and even into adulthood [7,8].

Different perinatal factors have also been related with subsequent respiratory morbidity in children born preterm; including bronchopulmonary dysplasia (BPD) [5,6,8–10], intrauterine growth restriction [10,11], male sex [10] and Afro-American ethnicity [10], as well as non-perinatal factors: mainly, lower lung function, generally expressed in lower values of forced expiratory volume in the first second (FEV1), at the age when the study was performed [6].

One study [12] on the differences in lung function between infants with BPD and healthy ones, showed that the infants with BDP who presented recurrent wheeze had significant reductions in forced expiratory flow at 25% of the forced vital capacity (FEF25), and increased residual volume (RV), as compared to the normal infants. Furthermore, even when they were compared to their counterparts without wheeze, those infants who had suffered BPD and wheeze had both RV as well as the ratio between RV and the total lung capacity (TLC) significantly higher.

On the other hand, at least three cohorts that recruited healthy newborns to study risk factors for asthma inception have found that low lung function in infants is a risk factor for subsequent asthma [13–15], which suggests a very early origin of the condition; and that pre- and peri-natal factors must play an important role.

To the best of our knowledge, the relationship between lung function in preterm infants and respiratory morbidity at later ages has not been previously studied. Our objective is to study if, among children born prematurely, low values of different lung function parameters measured in infancy are risk factors for wheezing at pre-school age.

2. Experimental Section

Methods

Study population: This is a retrospective study, carried out on ex-preterm newborns, (gestational age under 32 weeks), to whom lung function tests were administered at a corrected age of six months and who, at the time of a telephone survey were between three and nine years of age. Children were born between 2010 and 2016. The initial sample included 167 patients, of whom a total of 142 accepted to participate. Patients who required oxygen beyond postmenstrual week 36 were diagnosed.

Telephone survey: Parents of the patients answered, over the telephone, the core wheezing questionnaire of the International Study on Asthma and Allergy in Children (ISAAC) http://isaac.auckland.ac.nz/resources/tools.php?menu=tools1), validated internationally.

Infant lung function: The forced vital capacity (FVC), the forced expiratory volume at 0.5 sec ($FEV_{0.5}$), the forced expiratory flows at 75% and between 25%–75% of the FVC (FEF_{75} and FEF_{25-75}, respectively) and the ratio of $FEV_{0.5}/FVC$ were measured at a corrected mean age of 27.7 ± 1.94 weeks, from the maximum expiratory curves obtained by means of the Rapid Chest Compression with Pre-insufflation technique in accordance with the American Thoracic Society and the European Respiratory Society (ATS-ERS) recommendations [16]. The tests were performed with Master-Screen Baby Body Plethysmograph equipment (Jaëger®, Germany) and the pre-insufflation was by means of coupling the Neopuff neonatal resuscitator (Fisher & Paykel Healthcare®, New Zealand) with the face mask. All the infants were sedated with chloral hydrate at a dose of 80–100 mg/Kg and oxygen saturation was continually controlled using pulse oximetry.

Rehospitalizations due to respiratory causes: the number of admissions to hospital due to respiratory causes was obtained from review of the "Ágora" computer register of the Health Authority of Murcia, which records all admissions and their causes for all the population of the Region of Murcia, Spain. The policy regarding the use of Palivizumab, in our medium, is to administer it on the first day of life to all patients with BPD and to all the preterm newborns below 29 weeks of gestational age; thus, almost all the sample (96%) was treated.

Statistical study: To calculate the power of the study, a variance in the z-score of $FEV_{0.5}$ (0.76) found in this study has been considered. For a difference in the mean $FEV_{0.5}$ z-score of 0.5, a 95% confidence interval, and a power of ≥80%, required a total of 48 patients per group.

The association between qualitative variables was tested by means of the analysis of the contingency tables using Pearson's Chi-squared statistic. Student's t-test was used to compare the means of the quantitative variables.

Additionally, multivariate regression logistic analyses were carried out, with the presence of wheezing in the past (yes/no) being the dependent variable and including the following independent variables: age at time of survey; sex; attending day-care/school (yes/no); presence of BPD; gestational age (weeks); birthweight z-score; allergic mother (yes/no); and z-score of each of the lung function parameters (FVC, $FEV_{0.5}$, $FEV_{0.5}/FVC$, FEF_{75} and FEF_{25-75}) in different models: one model for each lung function parameter. The same analyses were performed considering exclusively wheeze in the past year (yes/no) as the dependent variable and with the same independent variables.

On the other hand, linear regression analyses were carried out, using the number of wheezing episodes as the dependent variable. The following were used as independent variables: age at time of survey; sex; attending day-care/school (yes/no); presence of BPD; gestational age (weeks); birthweight z-score; and allergic mother (yes/no). As in the previous case, the analyses were repeated including, as the independent variable, each of the results of the z-score of the lung function parameters, with a different model for each one.

The study was approved by the Ethics Committee of the Virgen de la Arrixaca University Hospital from Murcia (ethical approval code: 2007-1-1-HCUVA).

3. Results

From the initial sample, which included 167 patients, a total of 142 (85.03%) accepted to participate.

3.1. Wheezing Ever

Some 50% of the children studied presented wheeze at some point on their life (Table 1).

Table 1. Demographic characteristics, risk factors and lung function values and their differences between the children with or without ever wheezing.

	Total (142)	Wheezing: No (72)	Wheezing: Yes (70)	p *
Age (years)	5.37 (1.64)	5.22 (1.65)	5.53 (1.63)	0.27
Number of episodes	–	–	1.37 (0.65)	–
Gestational age (weeks)	27.7 (1.94)	27.76 (2.04)	27.77 (1.84)	0.98
Birthweight (g)	1034.3 (309)	1021.4 (287.6)	1047.6 (331.1)	0.62
Birthweight (z-score)	−0.33 (0.73)	−0.37 (0.79)	−0.28 (0.65)	0.47
Corrected age at test (months)	25.8 (15.7)	24.2 (16.4)	27.4 (14.8)	0.23
BPD	88 (62.0%)	38 (52.8%)	50 (71.4%)	0.022
Invasive ventilation	95 (66.9%)	48 (66.7%)	47 (67.1)	0.95
Day-care attendance in the first year	97 (68.3%)	46 (63.9%)	51 (72.9%)	0.25
Male sex	84 (59.2%)	44 (61.1%)	40 (57.1%)	0.63
Smoking during pregnancy	27 (19.3%)	11 (15.5%)	16 (23.2%)	0.25
FVC (z-score)	−1.12 (0.57)	−1.10 (0.63)	−1.14 (0.51)	0.72
$FEV_{0.5}$ (z-score)	−2.09 (0.87)	−1.94 (0.93)	−2.24 (0.79)	0.044
$FEV_{0.5}/FVC$ (z-score)	−0.45 (1.29)	−0.27 (1.36)	−0.62 (1.20)	0.11
FEF_{75} (z-score)	−1.47 (0.91)	−1.34 (0.93)	−1.61 (0.87)	0.07
FEF_{25-75} (z-score)	−1.54 (0.95)	−1.35 (0.97)	−1.73 (0.90)	0.02
Allergic mother	21 (15.2%)	5 (7%)	16 (23.9%)	0.008
Rehospitalisation due to respiratory causes	37 (18.4%)	13 (13.3%)	24 (23.3%)	0.06

Indicates number of cases (percentage) or mean (SD). * Difference between the proportion of children with wheezing according to each risk factor.

The univariate analysis showed that the presence of wheezing is associated with the z-score of different lung function measurements (FEV0.5, FEF75 and FEF25-75). The diagnosis of BPD constituted a consistent risk factor in all the multivariate analyses, independently of the lung function parameter included in it, with the OR value ranging from 2.45 (95% CI 1.07–5.63), $p = 0.03$ to 2.32 (95% CI 1.01–5.35), $p = 0.047$. Likewise, the mother having allergy also constituted a consistent risk factor in all the multivariate analyses, independently of the lung function parameter included in it, with the OR value ranging from 5.51 (95% CI 1.70–17.88), $p = 0.005$ to 4.94 (1.53–15.96), $p = 0.008$. The multivariate analysis showed that all the low lung function values analyzed, except FVC, were risk factors for wheezing at some time in their life (Figure 1).

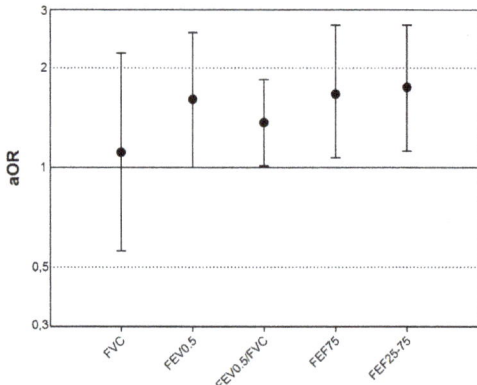

Figure 1. Risk of wheezing ever per z-score unit decrease of lung function. Adjusted odds ratios corrected for age, gender, daycare attendance, gestational age, birth weight (z-score), bronchopulmonary dysplasia, and allergic mother.

3.2. Wheezing in the Past Year

A total of 14.8% of the children studied presented wheezing in the past year (Table 2). There were statistically significant differences ($p = 0.013$) in the prevalence of wheezing between the patients with BPD (24.6%) and no-BPD (10.4%). The univariate analysis showed that the presence of wheezing in the past year was associated with the FEF25-75 z-score (-1.47 ± 0.95 vs. -1.93 ± 0.91; $p = 0.04$) (Table 2).

The multivariate analysis showed that all the lung function measurements analyzed, except FVC, were risk factors for wheezing in the past year (Figure 2), but suffering from BPD, although it showed a clear trend, was no longer a risk factor for wheezing in the past year (OR 2.46 (95% CI 1.07–5.63), $p = 0.03$ for the model that included FVC, but OR 3.16 (95% CI 0.89; 11.18) $p = 0.074$ in the model that included FEV05/FVC). The mother having an allergy also constituted a consistent risk factor in all the multivariate analyses, independently of the lung function parameter included therein, with the OR ranging from 7.66 (95% CI 1.67–35.04), $p = 0.009$ to 5.61 (1.39–22.67), $p = 0.015$.

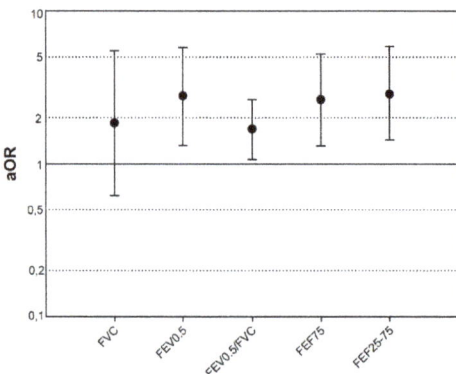

Figure 2. Risk of wheezing during the last year per z-score unit decrease of lung function. Adjusted odds ratios corrected for age, gender, daycare attendance, gestational age, birth weight (z-score), bronchopulmonary dysplasia, and allergic mother.

Table 2. Demographic characteristics, risk factors and lung function values and their differences between the children with or without wheezing in the last year.

	Total (142)	Wheezing in Last Year: No (121)	Wheezing in Last Year: Yes (21)	p *
Age (years)	5.37 (1.64)	5.47 (1.66)	4.81 (1.47)	0.09
Number of episodes	0.68 (0.82)	0.41 (0.51)	2.19 (0.6)	<0.001
Gestational age	27.77 (1.94)	27.75 (1.94)	27.86 (1.98)	0.82
Birthweight (g)	1034.3 (309)	1014.3 (295)	1149.9 (366)	0.06
Birthweight (z-score)	−0.33 (0.73)	−0.37 (0.74)	-0.07 (0.62)	0.07
Corrected age at test (sem.)	25.8 (15.7)	25.6 (16.4)	26.7 (11.1)	0.77
BPD (yes)	88 (62%)	72 (59.5%)	16 (76.2%)	0.15
Invasive ventilation (yes)	95 (66.9%)	15 (71.4%)	80 (66.1%)	0.80
Day-care attendance in first year	71 (72.5%)	54 (68.9%)	17 (89.5%)	0.06
Male sex	62 (63.3%)	52 (65.8%)	10 (52.6%)	0.28
Smoking during pregnancy	15 (15.8%)	11 (14.5%)	4 (21.1%)	0.49
FVC (z-score)	−1.12 (0.57)	−1.11 (0.60)	−1.18 (0.39)	0.6
$FEV_{0.5}$ (z-score)	−2.09 (0.87)	−2.04 (0.89)	−2.36 (0.72)	0.12
$FEV_{0.5}/FCV$ (z-score)	−0.45 (1.29)	−0.37 (1.30)	−0.89 (1.15)	0.09
FEF_{75} (z-score)	−1.47 (0.91)	−1.42 (0.90)	−1.79 (0.91)	0.08
FEF_{25-75} (z-score)	−1.54 (0.95)	−1.47 (0.95)	−1.93 (0.91)	0.04
Allergic mother (yes)	15 (16.3)	11 (14.9%)	4 (22.2%)	0.48
Rehospitalisation due to respiratory causes	36 (18.4%)	29 (17.9%)	8 (20.5%)	0.71

Indicates number of cases (percentage) or mean media (SD). * Difference between the proportion of children with wheezing according to each risk factor.

3.3. Number of Wheezing Episodes

On the other hand, the number of wheezing episodes referred by the parents was significantly greater in those children who still presented wheezing in the past year (2.19 ± 0.6 vs. 0.41 ± 0.51; $p < 0.001$). However, the multivariate analysis showed that the number of exacerbations was related with all of the lung function parameters analyzed, except FVC, and having an allergic mother (Table 3), but attending day-care in the first year of life was not (β coef.: 0.18; 95% CI -0.11 to 0.47; $p = 0.227$).

Table 3. List of number of episodes, referred by the parents, with different independent variables.

Variable	ß Coef. (95% CI)	p
FVC (z-score)	−0.073 (−0.33; 0.18)	0.575
$FEV_{0.5}$ (z-score)	−0.20 (−0.37; −0.04)	0.015
$FEV_{0.5}/FVC$ (z-score)	−0.13 (−0.23; −0.03)	0.015
FEF_{75} (z-score)	−0.21 (−0.36; −0.06)	0.007
FEF_{25-75} (z-score)	−0.22 (−0.36; −0.07)	0.003

3.4. Rehospitalisation Due to Respiratory Causes

The number of patients admitted to hospital for respiratory reasons was 27/140, which amounted to 19.29% (in two cases we do not have the data as the patients left the Region of Murcia). Of the children diagnosed with BPD, 20.9% were admitted to hospital on at least one occasion, compared to 16.7% of the preterm children without BPD ($p = 0.534$). No relationship was found between the variables studied and hospital admission or not due to respiratory causes. However, the multivariate analysis showed that a FEV0.5/FVC value lower than the lower limit of normality, was a risk factor for hospital admission (OR: 3.07; 95% CI 1.02 to 9.25; p = 0.046)

4. Discussion

In this study on the prevalence of wheezing in pre-school age children who had been born preterm, with or without BPD, almost half of them presented wheeze ever; however, only 21 out of 142 (14.8%) still presented wheeze in the past year, with the prevalence in children with BPD being slightly more than double as compared to those without BPD (18.2% vs. 9.2%). This prevalence is somewhat lower than the data published from the EPICURE study [6] on wheezing at 11 years of age in former very preterm children who, in the past year, 21% still had wheeze; although an additional 25% were diagnosed with asthma or were under treatment with asthma medication for respiratory symptoms. The children in that study had a mean age of 10.9 ± 0.38 years, significantly older than those in our sample (5.37 ± 1.64 years) and the percentage of patients with BPD was also higher in the EPICURE study (71% vs. 62%). In children between three and five years of age, the prevalence of wheezing was reported as 32% and 39%, respectively, in BDP and non-BDP patients (p = 0.51) [17]; however, the children in that study were born between 1998 and 2001, and our cohort were born between 2010 and 2016, which may explain the difference in prevalence. One study carried out in Germany [18], in a group of nine-year-old children who had been born preterm with a very similar gestational age to that of the present study, found a prevalence of wheezing of 14% and 4% in BDP and non-BDP patients, respectively, albeit without statistical significance, although this was probably due to the reduced size of the sample, which included only 28 patients in each group. It also corresponded to children born between 1994 and 2002; much earlier than our sample.

The respiratory morbidity of these former preterm infants is not only frequent, but also shows a potential severity, since almost 20% have been admitted to hospital, at least once in their lives, due to respiratory causes. We have found no significant differences in hospital admissions among those children diagnosed with BPD (20.9%) compared to those without (16.7%). The survey carried out by Vrijlandt et al. [17] referred to hospital admissions only in the first three months of life and found differences between BPD and non-BPD patients (54% vs. 14%; p < 0.001). The figures of rehospitalization in our study are, likewise, lower than those published by vom Hobe et al. [18] (36% and 21%, respectively). It is possible that the birth year of the children in each of the studies (the present one is later), as well as the use of palivizumab, systematic in our case and which is not reported in these two studies, can explain the lower number of patients admitted to hospital in our sample. Independently of the presence of BPD, in the total group, we found no association between hospital admittance and wheezing in the past year (18.9% vs. 21.6%; p = 0.706); although it almost reaches significance if we consider ever wheezing as opposed to never (64.9% vs. 35.1%; p = 0.06), probably as a consequence of those admitted due to bronchiolitis in the first year of life.

We have described for the first time, to the best of our knowledge, that infant lung function, essentially the obstructive pattern (FEV0.5/FVC) is a risk factor for respiratory morbidity: ever wheezing (Figure 1), wheezing in the past year (Figure 2) and also rehospitalization due to respiratory causes (FEV0.5/FVC < LLN: OR = 3.07; 95% CI 1.02 to 9.25; p = 0.046) in schoolchildren who were born preterm. It has been described that lung function in preterm children is lower with respect to their counterparts born at term, already in the infant stage [3] and that that alteration persists into school age [6] and even into adulthood [1]. Moreover, the preterm children who suffer BPD have a worse lung function than those born at term, during infancy [3,4], and even than the non-BPD preterm newborns [19], and this lost lung function, with regard to the healthy population, persists until school age [5,6] and even into adulthood [7,8]. The association of respiratory morbidity and alterations in lung function present at the moment of the survey or evaluation [7] has likewise been described, although not in all studies [2,6,18]. This would suggest that it is not only a structural reason which explains the respiratory morbidity, and that there must be other yet to be identified factors. For instance, in our case having an allergic mother is an independent risk factor for wheezing, although not for rehospitalization, which contradicts other publications that showed that family atopy is not a risk factor for wheezing among preterm children [2].

This study presents several limitations: firstly, the assessment of wheezing was carried out by means of a questionnaire and, although widely used throughout the world, this technique is always more subject to bias than if the assessment had been prospective. However, we believe that this bias cannot occur in the case of rehospitalization, given that the method used is the regional registry in which the clinical records of each patients are kept. Another limitation of the study is that no study of atopy had been performed in the patients; even more so if we consider that a relationship has been observed between maternal atopy and risk of wheeze. We do not really know how this information may have affected the results modifying the relationship between early lung function and subsequent wheezing, but it is probable that—as occurs with maternal allergy—this factor could have been independent of the best or worst early lung function. It would probably have modified the relationship between allergy in the mother and the higher prevalence of wheezing.

5. Conclusions

In conclusion, and apart from corroborating prior studies regarding the high prevalence of respiratory morbidity among children who were preterm newborns, we have found that the limitation in lung function at an infant age is a predictive factor both for subsequent wheezing and also for rehospitalisation.

Author Contributions: Conceptualization, M.S.-S.; methodology, M.S.-S.; validation, M.S.-S., L.G.-M., P.M.-L., and P.W.G.-M.; phone surveys, M.S.P.-C.; writing—original draft preparation, P.W.G.-M.; writing—review and editing, M.S.-S., M.S.P.-C., P.M.-L., P.W.G.-M., L.G.-M. All authors have read and agreed to the published version of the manuscript.

Funding: This research received no external funding.

Acknowledgments: In this section you can acknowledge any support given which is not covered by the author contribution or funding sections. This may include administrative and technical support, or donations in kind (e.g., materials used for experiments).

Conflicts of Interest: The authors declare no conflict of interest.

References

1. Sonnenschein-van der Voort, A.M.; Arends, L.R.; de Jongste, J.C.; Annesi-Maesano, I.; Arshad, S.H.; Barros, H.; Basterrechea, M.; Bisgaard, H.; Chatzi, L.; Corpeleijn, E.; et al. Preterm birth, infant weight gain, and childhood asthma risk: A meta-analysis of 147,000 European children. *J. Allergy Clin. Immunol.* **2014**, *133*, 1317–1329. [CrossRef] [PubMed]
2. Edwards, M.O.; Kotecha, S.J.; Lowe, J.; Richards, L.; Watkins, W.J.; Kotecha, S. Management of Prematurity-Associated Wheeze and Its Association with Atopy. *PLoS ONE* **2016**, *11*, e0155695. [CrossRef] [PubMed]
3. Friedrich, L.; Stein, R.T.; Pitrez, P.M.; Corso, A.L.; Jones, M.H. Reduced lung function in healthy preterm infants in the first months of life. *Am. J. Respir. Crit. Care Med.* **2006**, *173*, 442–447. [CrossRef] [PubMed]
4. Friedrich, L.; Pitrez, P.M.; Stein, R.T.; Goldani, M.; Tepper, R.; Jones, M.H. Growth rate of lung function in healthy preterm infants. *Am. J. Respir. Crit. Care Med.* **2007**, *176*, 1269–1273. [CrossRef] [PubMed]
5. Doyle, L.W.; Cheung, M.M.; Ford, G.W.; Olinsky, A.; Davis, M.N.; Callanan, C. Birth Weight <1501 G and Respiratory Health at Age 14. *Arch. Dis. Child.* **2001**, *84*, 40–44. [CrossRef] [PubMed]
6. Fawke, J.; Lum, S.; Kirkby, J.; Hennessy, E.; Marlow, N.; Rowell, V.; Thomas, S.; Stocks, J. Lung function and respiratory symptoms at 11 years in children born extremely preterm: The EPICure study. *Am. J. Respir. Crit. Care Med.* **2010**, *182*, 237–245. [CrossRef] [PubMed]
7. Den Dekker, H.T.; Sonnenschein-van der Voort, A.M.M.; de Jongste, J.C.; Anessi-Maesano, I.; Arshad, S.H.; Barros, H.; Beardsmore, C.S.; Bisgaard, H.; Phar, S.C.; Craig, L.; et al. Early growth characteristics and the risk of reduced lung function and asthma: A meta-analysis of 25,000 children. *J. Allergy Clin. Immunol.* **2016**, *137*, 1026–1035. [CrossRef] [PubMed]

8. Kotecha, S.J.; Edwards, M.O.; Watkins, W.J.; Henderson, A.J.; Paranjothy, S.; Dunstan, F.D.; Kotecha, S. Effect of preterm birth on later FEV1: A systematic review and meta-analysis. *Thorax* **2013**, *68*, 760–766. [CrossRef] [PubMed]
9. Evans, M.; Palta, M.; Sadek, M.; Weinstein, M.R.; Peters, M.E. Associations between Family History of Asthma, Bronchopulmonary Dysplasia, and Childhood Asthma in Very Low Birth Weight Children. *Am. J. Epidemiol.* **1998**, *148*, 460–466. [CrossRef] [PubMed]
10. Keller, R.L.; Feng, R.; DeMauro, S.B.; Ferkol, T.; Hardie, W.; Rogers, E.E.; Stevens, T.P.; Voynow, J.A.; Bellamy, S.L.; Shaw, P.A.; et al. Prematurity and Respiratory Outcomes Program. Bronchopulmonary Dysplasia and Perinatal Characteristics Predict 1-Year Respiratory Outcomes in Newborns Born at Extremely Low Gestational Age: A Prospective Cohort Study. *J. Pediatr.* **2017**, *187*, 89–97. [CrossRef] [PubMed]
11. Kindlund, K.; Thomsen, S.F.; Stensballe, L.G.; Skytthe, A.; Kyvik, O.; Backer, V.; Bisgaard, H. Birth Weight and Risk of Asthma in 3-9-year-old Twins: Exploring the Fetal Origins Hypothesis. *Thorax* **2010**, *65*, 146–149. [CrossRef] [PubMed]
12. Robin, B.; Kim, Y.J.; Huth, J.; Klocksieben, J.; Torres, M.; Tepper, R.S.; Castile, R.G.; Solway, J.; Hershenson, M.; Goldstein-Filbrun, A. Pulmonary Function in Bronchopulmonary Dysplasia. *Pediatr. Pulmonol.* **2004**, *37*, 236–242. [CrossRef] [PubMed]
13. Bisgaard, H.; Jensen, S.M.; Bønnelykke, K. Interaction between asthma and lung function growth in early life. *Am. J. Respir. Crit. Care Med.* **2012**, *185*, 1183–1189. [CrossRef] [PubMed]
14. Brooke, E.; Lucas, J.S.; Collins, S.A.; Holloway, J.W.; Roberts, G.; Inskip, H.; Godfrey, K.M.; Cooper, C.; Pike, K.C.; Southampton Women's Survey Study Group. Infant lung function and wheeze in later childhood in the Southampton Women's Survey. *Eur. Respir. J.* **2014**, *43*, 919–921. [CrossRef] [PubMed]
15. Pike, K.C.; Rose-Zerilli, M.J.; Osvald, E.C.; Inskip, H.M.; Godfrey, K.M.; Crozier, S.R.; Roberts, G.; Clough, J.B.; Holloway, J.W.; Lucas, J.S.; et al. The relationship between infant lung function and the risk of wheeze in the preschool years. *Pediatr. Pulmonol.* **2011**, *46*, 75–82. [CrossRef] [PubMed]
16. Lum, S.; Stocks, J.; Castile, R.; Davis, S. ATS/ERS Statement: Raised Volume Forced Expirations in Infants: Guidelines for Current Practice. *Am. J. Respir. Crit. Care Med* **2005**, *172*, 1463–1471.
17. Vrijlandt, E.J.; Boezen, H.M.; Gerritsen, J.; Stremmelaar, E.F.; Duiverman, E.J. Respiratory health in prematurely born preschool children with and without bronchopulmonary dysplasia. *J. Pediatr.* **2007**, *150*, 256–261. [CrossRef] [PubMed]
18. Vom Hove, M.; Prenzel, F.; Uhlig, H.H.; Robel-Tillig, E.R. Pulmonary Outcome in Former Preterm, Very Low Birth Weight Children with Bronchopulmonary Dysplasia: A Case-Control Follow-Up at School Age. *J. Pediatr.* **2014**, *164*, 40–45. [CrossRef] [PubMed]
19. Sanchez-Solis, M.; Perez-Fernandez, V.; Bosch-Gimenez, V.; Quesada, J.J.; Garcia-Marcos, L. Lung function gain in preterm infants with and without bronchopulmonary dysplasia. *Pediatr. Pulmonol.* **2016**, *51*, 936–942. [CrossRef] [PubMed]

Publisher's Note: MDPI stays neutral with regard to jurisdictional claims in published maps and institutional affiliations.

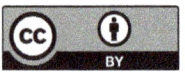

© 2020 by the authors. Licensee MDPI, Basel, Switzerland. This article is an open access article distributed under the terms and conditions of the Creative Commons Attribution (CC BY) license (http://creativecommons.org/licenses/by/4.0/).

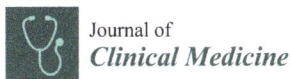

Article

The Role of Airways 17β-Estradiol as a Biomarker of Severity in Postmenopausal Asthma: A Pilot Study

Giulia Scioscia [1,2], Giovanna Elisiana Carpagnano [3], Donato Lacedonia [1,2,*], Piera Soccio [1,2], Carla Maria Irene Quarato [1], Luigia Trabace [4], Paolo Fuso [1] and Maria Pia Foschino Barbaro [1,2]

1. Department of Medical and Surgical Sciences, University of Foggia, 71122 Foggia, Italy; giulia.scioscia@unifg.it (G.S.); piera.soccio@unifg.it (P.S.); carlamariairene.quarato@gmail.com (C.M.I.Q.); paolo.fuso91@gmail.com (P.F.); mariapia.foschino@unifg.it (M.P.F.B.)
2. Institute of Respiratory Diseases, Policlinico Riuniti of Foggia, 71122 Foggia, Italy
3. Department of Basic Medical Sciences, Neuroscience and Sense Organs, Section of Respiratory Disease, University "Aldo Moro" of Bari, 70121 Bari, Italy; elisiana.carpagnano@uniba.it
4. Department of Clinical and Sperimental Medicine, University of Foggia, 71122 Foggia, Italy; luigia.trabace@unifg.it
* Correspondence: donato.lacedonia@unifg.it; Tel.: +39-0881733084

Received: 15 May 2020; Accepted: 27 June 2020; Published: 29 June 2020

Abstract: Background: Asthma severity differs according to gender; in adult women, there is higher prevalence and severity of asthma than in men, and it coincides with changes in sex hormones. Recently, a new phenotype of asthma has been identified that appears after menopause, and it may be associated with decreased estrogen levels. Our goal was to study the 17β-estradiol (E2) concentrations in the blood and airways of women affected by asthma onset after menopause, evaluating its possible role in the severity of the disease. Methods: We enrolled 33 consecutive women with a diagnosis of postmenopausal asthma, recruited from the outpatient pulmonary clinic: 18 with severe (SA) and 15 with mild-to-moderate (MMA) asthma. We also included 30 age-matched healthy menopausal women as controls (HS). All subjects enrolled underwent blood and sputum collection (IS), and E2 concentrations were determined in plasma and sputum supernatant samples using an enzyme-linked immunosorbent assay (ELISA) kit. Results: Significantly higher serum concentrations of E2 were found in postmenopausal SA compared to MMA and HS, respectively (33 ± 5.5 vs. 24 ± 6.63 vs. 7.79 ± 1.54 pg/mL, $p < 0.05$). Similar results were found in the IS: significantly higher levels of E2 were detected in patients with postmenopausal SA compared with MMA and HS, respectively (0.34 ± 0.17 vs. 0.26 ± 0.13 vs. 0.07 ± 0.06 pg/mL, $p < 0.05$). We found positive correlations between IS E2 concentrations and sputum neutrophil levels in SA group ($\rho = 0.52$, $p < 0.05$). Conclusions: Our findings showed the possibility to measure E2 in the airways, and it has increased in postmenopausal asthmatic patients, especially in those with SA. Airways E2 levels may serve as a suitable biomarker of postmenopausal SA to help to phenotype SA patients with neutrophil inflammation.

Keywords: estradiol; severe asthma; postmenopausal asthma; sputum

1. Introduction

Gender differences in the incidence, prevalence and severity of asthma are reported by epidemiological data. These differences also change throughout life. During childhood, the prevalence of asthma shows a higher risk in boys compared to girls. Otherwise, after puberty, there is an increase of asthma incidence in women until menopause [1,2]. The causes of gender differences are unknown; however, the hypothesis of the possible link between the higher incidence of asthma in women and changes in sex hormones was evaluated.

Three types of estrogen molecules are produced in human females: estradiol, estrone and estriol. Estradiol is the major female sex hormone, and its levels are predominant during a woman's reproductive years. Conversely, during the menopausal period, the amount of estradiol declines to very low levels. Moreover, in pregnant women, there is a large amount of estriol, while estrone becomes predominant in menopause.

Recent studies proved that estrogen increases the T helper (Th) 2 response in the presence of allergens, likely by stimulating the proliferation and differentiation of Th cells into Th2 cells [3].

Another mechanism is that the presence of physiologic concentrations of 17β-estradiol seem to induce mast cells' degranulation and to enhance allergen crosslinking with surface IgE [4,5]. On the other hand, testosterone has been shown to attenuate type 2 innate lymphoid cells' (ILC2) function and proliferation [6].

Estradiol may increase the release of IL-1β and TNF-α and, at the same time, decrease the release of IL-10, promoting inflammation [7]. Instead, progesterone may cause eosinophilia, as it significantly increases the IL-10, IL1-β and TNF-α amounts in the lungs and the release of IL-4 by bone marrow cells [8].

Women with severe asthma also showed a higher IL-23R expression and IL-17A production by Th17-differentiated cells when compared with severely asthmatic men [9]. A similar molecular environment was reproduced in ovariectomized mice receiving 17β-estradiol [9].

A new phenotype of asthma with onset after menopause has been recently described for a subset of women [10,11], but the mechanisms that initiate and regulate postmenopausal asthma remain largely unknown. Among women over 50 years of age, menopause can either coincide with the onset of asthma or be associated with the deterioration of a preexisting asthma condition [11]. After menopause, estrogen levels decrease to the levels observed in patients with surgical oophorectomy, who also show extremely low progesterone levels. The incidence of asthma may be associated with the abrupt decrease in estrogen levels and the consequent impairment in the hypothalamic-pituitary-gonadal axis that occurs during the menopausal transition.

Menopausal-onset asthma affects 18% of the total female asthma population, and frequently, it is characterized by the absence of atopy; recurrent sinusitis; aspirin sensitivity and/or intolerance to angiotensin-converting enzyme inhibitors, greater severity (use of systemic steroids to control symptoms and frequent hospitalizations) and an altered perception of asthmatic symptoms [11,12].

All sex steroid hormone receptors were found in the lungs: estrogen receptor (ER-α or ER-β), progesterone receptor (PR-A or PR-B) and an androgen receptor (AR). The activation of steroid hormones occurs as a result of the link with their own unique receptors. Among different estrogens, estradiol is the one having the greatest affinity for estrogen receptors and the same binding affinity for both ER-α and ER-β [8].

Sex hormone-binding globulin (SHBG) is an important steroid hormone binding protein in human plasma and regulates sex hormone delivery to tissues and cells by binding them and keeping them inactive.

Under normal conditions, in the blood stream, testosterone (T) and 17β-estradiol (E2) are largely bound to SHBG. Instead, a smaller part (~2%) is dissociated from SHBG, and the nonbound hormone is the biologically active fraction [13].

The aim of our study was to analyze the blood and airways' E2 concentrations of women affected by asthma onset after menopause, evaluating its possible role in the severity of the disease and comparing it with other inflammatory biomarkers.

2. Methods

2.1. Patients

Thirty-three consecutive women with postmenopausal asthma, 18 with severe and 15 with mild-to-moderate asthma, were recruited in this study from the outpatient facility of the Institute of Respiratory Disease of the University of Foggia, Italy. We also enrolled 30 age-matched healthy menopausal women as controls. Written informed consent was obtained from all subjects, and the study was approved by the institutional ethics committee of the University of Foggia (institutional review board approval No. 17/CE/2014).

All women were classified as postmenopausal on the basis of a completed questionnaire to confirm whether or not they had entered menopause (cessation of menstruation for 12 months). They were considered to be postmenopausal asthmatics if their asthma had started at menopause, i.e., in the period between 1 year before and 1 year after their last menstrual period. All patients with asthma were assessed within a period of stability and at least 4 weeks after an upper respiratory tract infection and were classified and treated according to Global Initiative for Asthma (GINA) guidelines [14]. Smokers, women on postmenopausal hormone replacement therapy (HRT) and asthmatics randomized in a controlled trial and/or with biologic therapy were excluded from the study.

At the first visit, a complete baseline questionnaire requesting information on medical history, menopausal status, hormone use and other reproductive and lifestyle variables was administered to all subjects. Subsequently, they received a physical examination, including body mass index (BMI) measurement, atopy assessment, exhaled nitric oxide (FENO) measurement and spirometry with a bronchial obstruction reversibility test. During the second visit, subjects underwent blood analysis for serum levels of E2 and cells count and, finally, sputum induction (IS). Hormones were dosed after a standardized rest, at the same time of day for all subjects, as they are known to be extremely dependent on circadian rhythm, stress, treatments, etc.

2.2. Menopausal Assessment

The menopausal status was assessed by a standardized self-administered questionnaire. All the participants were asked to indicate their putative mean menopause age and whether it was natural or surgical. In the case of physiological menopause, they were asked to enlist the date of their last period; otherwise, they were asked to indicate type, reason and date of surgical intervention. The women were also inquired about their medical history, with specific questions investigating about any concomitant state and relative treatment of conditions that may mimic menopausal symptoms, including depression, anemia, hypothyroidism, diabetes, previous contraceptives uses and concurrent hormone replacement therapy (HRT). As an exclusion criterion, women in concurrent HRT were not enrolled in the study. The last item of the questionnaire concerned the onset of asthma symptoms, also investigating if any respiratory symptoms had ever been previously experimented in conjunction with the menstrual cycle or eventual pregnancies. In the case of doubts about a preexisting asthma worsened at menopause, patients were excluded from the study too.

2.3. Atopic Status

All the enrolled subjects were skin prick-tested, and the atopic status was assessed as SPOT positiveness. Skin prick tests (SPTs) were performed using a standard panel for common aeroallergens (Lofarma, Italy) [15].

2.4. Lung Function

Pulmonary function tests were performed. Forced expiratory volume in one second (FEV1), forced vital capacity (FVC) and plethysmographic lung volumes were measured using a spirometer (Sensormedics, Milan, Italy) following international standards in all subjects [16,17]. The best value of three maneuvers was expressed as a percentage of the predicted normal value. After the baseline evaluation, spirometry was repeated 15 min after the subjects had inhaled 400 mg of salbutamol, as previously reported. The reversibility of airways obstruction was expressed in terms of the percent changes from the baseline of FEV1.

2.5. Measurement of FENO

The Medisoft FENO+ device (Medisoft Belgium, Sorinnes, Belgium), which is a semiportable for repeatable multiflow measurements of exhaled NO with offline measurements, was used. It has a software package that provides step-by-step online quality control. The measurement range is 0–600 ppb. FENO was measured using a previously described restricted breath technique, which employed expiratory resistance and positive mouth pressure to close the velum and exclude nasal NO; expiratory flow measurements at 50 mL/s and a 350 mL/s have been evaluated. Repeated exhalations were performed until three plateaus agreed within 5% [18].

2.6. IS Collection and Processing

According to the method described by Toungoussova et al. [19], sputum was induced through the inhalation of hypertonic saline solution (4.5%) with an ultrasonic nebulizer (DeVilbiss Healthcare GmbH, Mannheim, Germany) and analyzed after the selection of mucus plugs. In patients with severe asthma, we used spontaneous sputum when they were particularly uncontrolled. Ten healthy subjects, 9 patients with severe asthma and 5 with mild-to-moderate asthma, were not able to produce adequate sputum samples (defined as containing at least 500 non-squamous cells), and their samples were discarded. The sputum (spontaneous or induced) was used for cytologic analysis, and the supernatant was used for E2 analysis.

2.7. 17-β-estradiol (E2) Analysis

A venous blood sample was drawn from each participant between 8 a.m. and 10 a.m., and the serum was obtained by centrifugation. Serum aliquots were then stored at $-80\,°C$ until analysis. The E2 concentration was determined in plasma and sputum supernatant samples using an enzyme-linked immunosorbent assay kit (Estradiol Serum EIA KIT, catalog number KB30-H1, Arbor Assays, Ann Arbor, MI, USA) as described in the manufacturer's instructions. Intra and interassay coefficients of variation were 4.1% and 9.6%, respectively.

2.8. Statistical Analysis

Descriptive statistics (i.e., means, standard deviations and percentages) were applied to summarize the continuous and categorical variables. One-way ANOVA and Kruskal–Wallis rank tests were used to compare groups. Correlation between variables was measured using the Spearman rank correlation test. Significance was defined as a p-value of <0.05. SPSS 22.0 (III INC, Chicago, IL, USA) was used to store and analyze the data.

3. Results

Anthropometric, clinical, functional and biologic data of subjects enrolled are reported in Table 1.

Table 1. Baseline characteristics of the study population.

Number of Patients	HS 30	MMA 15	SA 18
Demographic and clinical characteristics			
Age, years (mean ± SD)	62 ± 5.45	55 ± 18	58 ± 11
BMI, Kg/m^2, (mean ± SD)	27 ± 5	26 ± 5	28 ± 5
Age of onset, years (mean ± SD)		45 ± 8	40 ± 15
Postmenopausal status (%)	25 (83%)	12 (80%)	14 (78%)
Surgical menopause (%)	5 (17%)	3 (20%)	4 (22%)
Exacerbations/year, (mean ± SD)		1 ± 1 *	3 ± 1 *
Atopy (SPT+), n (%)	0 (0%)	5 (33.3%)	7 (38.8%)
Aspirin-sensitivity, n (%)		8 (53.3%)	10 (55.5%)
ICS low to medium dose, n (%)		12 (80%)	0
ICS high dose/LABA, n (%)		3 (20%) *	7 (38.8%) *
ICS high dose/LABA/TIOTROPIUM, n (%)		0	11 (61.1%)

Table 1. Cont.

Number of Patients	HS 30	MMA 15	SA 18
OCS, n (%)		0	10 (55.5%)
ACT		19 ± 3 *	14 ± 4 *
ACQ		1 ± 0.7 *	3 ± 2 *
Lung function			
FEV1 preBD, % predicted	85 ± 5 [†,¥]	78 ± 14 [*,¥]	67 ± 19 [†,*]
FEV_1/FVC preBD, %	82 ± 12 [†,¥]	68 ± 10 [¥]	62 ± 12 [†]
Reversibility, %	5 ± 4.5 [†,¥]	13 ± 9 [¥]	11 ± 6 [†]
TLC, % predicted	104 ± 13	98 ± 14	96 ± 14
RV, % predicted	89 ± 20	97 ± 25	110 ± 26
Biomarkers			
$FENO_{50}$, ppb	15 ± 6 [†,¥]	22 ± 28 [¥]	25 ± 21 [†]
Blood eosinophil count, cells/mL	0.05 ± 0.22 [†,¥]	0.21 ± 0.24 [¥]	0.25 ± 0.25 [†]
Blood neutrophil level, cells/mL	2.2 ± 1.7 [†]	2.7 ± 1.4 *	5.6 ± 2.7 [†,*]
Eosinophil IS count, % total cells	1 ± 1 [†,¥]	2 ± 2 [¥]	3 ± 2 [†]
Neutrophil IS level, % total cells	38 ± 18 [†]	37 ± 12 *	68 ± 15 [†,*]
Serum 17β-estradiol, pg/mL	7.79 ± 1.54 [†,¥]	24 ± 6.63 [*,¥]	33 ± 5.5 [†,*]
SEI 17β-estradiol, pg/mL	0.07 ± 0.06 [†,¥]	0.26 ± 0.13 [*,¥]	0.34 ± 0.17 [†,*]

Abbreviations. HS: healthy subjects, MMA: mild-moderate asthma, SA: severe asthma, BMI: body mass index, SPT+: SPOT positiveness, ICS: inhaled corticosteroids, ICS/LABA: inhaled corticosteroids/long-acting beta-adrenoceptor agonists, OCS: Oral Corticosteroids, ACT: asthma control test, ACQ: asthma control questionnaire, FEV1: forced expiratory volume, FEV1/FVC: forced expiratory volume/forced vital capacity, BD: Bronchodilator, FEF: forced expiratory flow, Raw: airway resistance, TLC: total lung capacity, RV: residual volume, RV/TLC: residual volume/total lung capacity, IS: induced sputum and SEI: induced sputum supernatant. [†] $p < 0.05$ between HS and SA, * $p < 0.05$ between SA and MMA and [¥] $p < 0.05$ between HS and MMA.

Higher serum concentrations of E2 were found in postmenopausal SA compared to MMA ones and healthy women (33 ± 5.5 vs. 24 ± 6.63 vs. 7.79 ± 1.54 pg/mL, $p < 0.05$) (Figure 1).

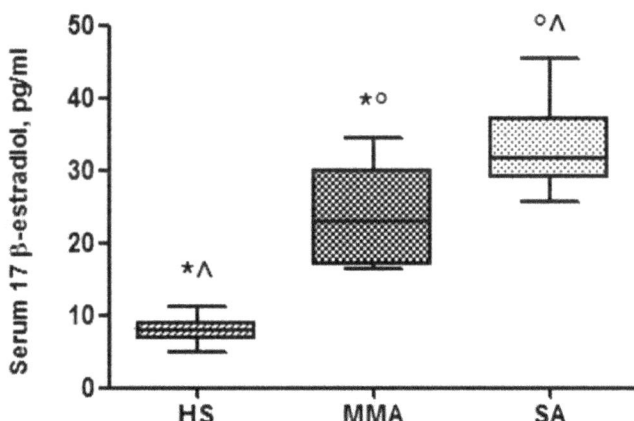

Figure 1. Serum concentrations of 17β-estradiol in healthy subjects (HS), mild-to-moderate asthma (MMA) and severe asthma (SA) groups. * $p < 0.05$ HS vs. MMA, ^ $p < 0.05$ HS vs. SA and ° $p < 0.05$ MMA vs. SA.

We found that E2 was detectable in all IS supernatant samples collected: 9 patients with SA, 10 patients with MMA and 20 HS. Similar results were found in the IS; i.e., significantly higher levels of E2 were found in patients with postmenopausal SA compared to MMA and HS, respectively (0.34 ± 0.17 vs. 0.26 ± 0.13 vs. 0.07 ± 0.06 pg/mL, $p < 0.05$) (Figure 2).

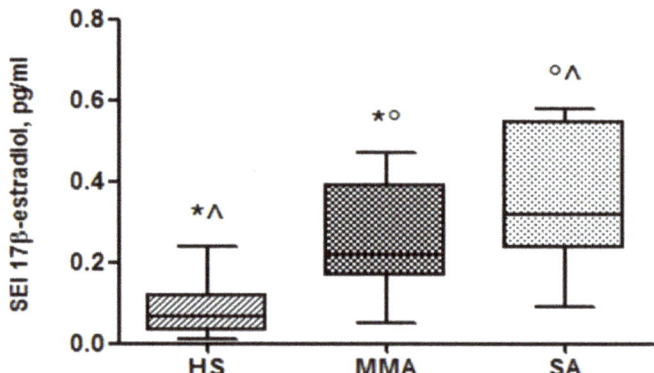

Figure 2. Induced sputum supernatant (SEI) concentrations of 17β-estradiol in HS, MMA and SA groups. * $p < 0.05$ HS vs. MMA, ^ $p < 0.05$ HS vs. SA and ° $p < 0.05$ MMA vs. SA.

In patients with postmenopausal SA, we found a positive correlation between IS E2 and neutrophil IS levels ($\rho = 0.52$, $p < 0.05$).

We did not find a significant correlation between serum and IS E2 levels and any correlations between serum and IS E2 with other clinical variables, such as BMI, ACT and ACQ scores, FEV1 and FENO.

4. Discussion

The main findings of this study were (1) the identification of higher serum concentrations of E2 in postmenopausal SA patients than in MMA and healthy menopausal ones, (2) for the first time, to our knowledge, the detection of E2 free levels in IS supernatants with higher concentrations in SA patients than MMA and HS, like in the serum samples and (3) the presence of a positive correlation of IS levels of E2 with IS neutrophils counted in the SA group.

Several studies aimed to understand the role of sex hormones in lung inflammatory processes [20]. Asthma is a chronic inflammatory disease characterized by a sexual dimorphism. In older adults, two phenotypes are usually observed: patients with long-standing asthma who develop additional airflow limitations and those who develop late-onset asthma [21].

During the menopausal period, the decline in sex hormones synthesis causes a loss of the hypothalamic feedback inhibition and a marked increase in gonadotropin-releasing hormone (GnRH) levels. However, data from a research study showed lower serum FSH and LH levels in menopausal women with new-onset asthma or preexisting lung disease compared to nonasthmatic postmenopausal women [22]. Furthermore, patients with secretion dysfunctions of cortical hormones have shown a more severe asthmatic phenotype characterized by repeated asthma attacks; these patients become more dependent on exogenous glucocorticoids [23].

These findings could justify the higher serum levels of E2 in postmenopausal SA patients than in MMA and healthy menopausal ones.

Under normal conditions, in the blood stream, testosterone (T) and 17β-estradiol (E2) are largely bound to SHBG. Instead, a smaller part (~2%) is dissociate from SHBG [13].

The 20–40% of circulating E2 is bound to SHBG that controls the sex hormone transport to tissues and cells. According to the free hormone hypothesis, the unbound quota is biologically active and freely diffuses across the cell surface membranes [24]. For the first time, in our pilot study, we detected E2 free levels in the IS supernatants, and the preliminary results confirm that menopausal SA shows higher concentrations than MMA and healthy menopausal subjects, regardless of the sputum collection method (spontaneous or induced). Indeed, the difference between the spontaneous or induced sputum is only in the collection's method, the latter being conducted by the help of the inhalation of a nebulized sterile saline solution (isotonic or hypertonic). Sputum cellular compositions and protein marker detections are not influenced by the method of collection, as previously reported by other studies in the literature [25].

We did not find a correlation between the serum and IS samples, probably due to the small number of patients.

Studies have shown that sex hormones can regulate airway inflammations, and estrogen increased Th2-mediated airway inflammations, although these effects are still under investigation.

Type 2 inflammation in asthma occurs in many patients but not all. In some patients with asthma is found an increase of IL-17A that seems associated with more severe forms of asthma [26]. CD4+ T helper, 17 (Th17) cells, γδ T cells, neutrophils and innate lymphoid cells are able to produce IL-17A in the lungs.

Newcomb DC et al. [9] found an increased production of IL-17A from Th17 cells in severe asthmatics women compared to men. Moreover, using a mouse model, the same authors showed that a rise of IL-17A is associated with an increased neutrophilic airway inflammation in female mice compared to male mice when stimulated by E2.

Consistent with the literature, we demonstrated a positive correlation between IS E2 and neutrophil IS levels in patients with postmenopausal SA, and our results confirm that neutrophils are considered to be central to the pathogenesis of most forms of severe late-onset asthma.

Nevertheless, more studies are needed to better understand the role of sex hormones in IL-17A-mediated airway inflammation and neutrophilic asthma.

Estrogens are shown to possess the ability to inhibit the chemotactic activity of polymorphonuclear leukocytes; on the contrary, progesterone increases it [27]. Furthermore, progesterone and testosterone may reduce the ROS and NO generation driven by estradiol [28,29]. Therefore, increased levels of E2 in the respiratory tract might fix neutrophils to the lower airway epithelium and give rise to local oxidative stress.

Additionally, in studies on human leukocytes, it has been shown that estrogens reduce the process of programmed cell death (i.e., apoptosis), while testosterone seems to favor it. This could allow the survival of self-reactive cells and, at least in part, explain the greater predisposition of women for Th17 and Th1-driven autoimmune diseases, such as rheumatoid arthritis (RA) and systemic lupus erythematosus (SLE) [30].

Gender-specific asthma pathogenesis may also be confounded by other comorbidities. The Severe Asthma Research Program (SARP) and the European Network for Understanding Mechanisms of Severe Asthma showed a higher body mass index (BMI) and neutrophilic inflammation among women with severe asthma compared to nonsevere asthma but not in men [31,32]. Additionally, in our study, female patients with severe asthma showed a slightly higher, if not statistically significant, BMI compared to those with mild-moderate asthma. Additionally, whether or not gender dimorphism is related to female hormones remains unclear. One possible explanation for the obese-asthma neutrophilic phenotype may be related to serum levels of leptin, a key player in body weight regulation, which increases helper T cell type 1 (Th1) inflammation [33]. However, several studies have shown a strong correlation between BMI and nonatopic asthma only in women of childbearing age and not in men. On the contrary, no gender difference has been reported in the incidence of atopic asthma [34,35]. Taken together, these data suggest the possibility of an interaction between gender, age, BMI and asthma type (atopic vs. nonatopic) in the pathogenesis of severe asthma in females.

The strengths of our preliminary study are the detection of E2 free levels in the IS supernatants of asthmatic patients and healthy controls and the study of clinical and inflammatory characteristics of a well-described phenotype that is postmenopausal asthma.

However, the study also has key limitations, such as the small number of subjects enrolled and the absence of a validation of E2 free levels detection technique in the sputum.

5. Conclusions

In conclusion, this preliminary study suggests that E2 plays a role in postmenopausal severe asthma. This hormone is detectable directly in the airways, and it may be a noninvasive marker to phenotype SA patients not eligible for actual biologic treatments with neutrophilic inflammation.

Author Contributions: Conceptualization, G.S. and D.L.; methodology, G.S., D.L. and G.E.C.; formal analysis P.S., C.M.I.Q. and P.F.; data curation, G.S., D.L. and P.S.; writing—Original draft preparation, G.S. and D.L.; writing—Review and editing, G.S., D.L., G.E.C., L.T. and M.P.F.B. and supervision, M.P.F.B. All authors have read and agreed to the published version of the manuscript.

Funding: This research did not receive any specific grant from funding agencies in the public, commercial or not-for-profit sectors.

Conflicts of Interest: The authors declare that they have no conflict of interest.

References

1. Fuseini, H.; Newcomb, D.C. Mechanisms Driving Gender Differences in Asthma. *Curr. Allergy Asthma Rep.* **2017**, *17*, 19. [CrossRef]
2. Zein, J.G.; Denson, J.L.; Wechsler, M.E. Asthma over the Adult Life Course: Gender and Hormonal Influences. *Clin. Chest Med.* **2019**, *40*, 149–161. [CrossRef]
3. Uemura, Y.; Liu, T.Y.; Narita, Y.; Suzuki, M.; Matsushita, S. 17β-Estradiol (E2) plus tumor necrosis factor-α induces a distorted maturation of human monocyte-derived dendritic cells and promotes their capacity to initiate T-helper 2 responses. *Hum. Immunol.* **2008**, *69*, 149–157. [CrossRef] [PubMed]
4. Zaitsu, M.; Narita, S.I.; Lambert, K.C.; Grady, J.J.; Estes, D.M.; Curran, E.M.; Brooks, E.G.; Watson, C.S.; Goldblum, R.M.; Midoro-Horiuti, T. Estradiol activates mast cells via a non-genomic estrogen receptor-α and calcium influx. *Mol. Immunol.* **2007**, *44*, 1977–1985. [CrossRef] [PubMed]
5. Bonds, R.S.; Midoro-Horiuti, T. Estrogen effects in allergy and asthma. *Curr. Opin. Allergy Clin. Immunol.* **2013**, *13*, 92–99. [CrossRef] [PubMed]
6. Cephus, J.Y.; Stier, M.T.; Fuseini, H.; Yung, J.A.; Toki, S.; Bloodworth, M.H.; Zhou, W.; Goleniewska, K.; Zhang, J.; Garon, S.L.; et al. Testosterone Attenuates Group 2 Innate Lymphoid Cell-Mediated Airway Inflammation. *Cell Rep.* **2017**, *21*, 2487–2499. [CrossRef]
7. de Oliveira, A.P.; Domingos, H.V.; Cavriani, G.; Damazo, A.S.; dos Santos Franco, A.L.; Oliani, S.M.; Oliveira-Filho, R.M.; Vargaftig, B.B.; de Lima, W.T. Cellular recruitment and cytokine generation in a rat model of allergic lung inflammation are differentially modulated by progesterone and estradiol. *Am. J. Physiol. Cell Physiol.* **2007**, *293*, C1120–C1128. [CrossRef] [PubMed]
8. Tam, A.; Morrish, D.; Wadsworth, S.; Dorscheid, D.; Man, S.P.; Sin, D.D. The role of female hormones on lung function in chronic lung diseases. *BMC Womens Health* **2011**, *11*, 24. [CrossRef] [PubMed]
9. Newcomb, D.C.; Cephus, J.Y.; Boswell, M.G.; Fahrenholz, J.M.; Langley, E.W.; Feldman, A.S.; Zhou, W.; Dulek, D.E.; Goleniewska, K.; Woodward, K.B.; et al. Estrogen and progesterone decrease let-7f microRNA expression and increase IL-23/IL-23 receptor signaling and IL-17A production in patients with severe asthma. *J. Allergy Clin. Immunol.* **2015**, *136*, 1025–1034. [CrossRef]
10. Balzano, G.; Fuschillo, S.; De Angelis, E.; Gaudiosi, C.; Mancini, A.; Caputi, M. Persistent airway inflammation and high exacerbation rate in asthma that starts at menopause. *Monaldi Arch. Chest Dis = Arch. Monaldi per le Mal del Torace* **2007**, *67*, 135–141. [CrossRef]
11. Foschino Barbaro, M.P.; Costa, V.R.; Resta, O.; Prato, R.; Spanevello, A.; Palladino, G.P.; Martinelli, D.; Carpagnano, G.E. Menopausal asthma: A new biological phenotype? *Allergy* **2010**, *65*, 1306–1312. [CrossRef] [PubMed]
12. Baldaçara, R.P.; Silva, I. Association between asthma and female sex hormones. *Sao Paulo Med. J.* **2017**, *135*, 4–14. [CrossRef] [PubMed]
13. De Ronde, W.; Van Der Schouw, Y.T.; Muller, M.; Grobbee, D.E.; Gooren, L.J.; Pols, H.A.; De Jong, F.H. Associations of Sex-Hormone-Binding Globulin (SHBG) with Non-SHBG-Bound Levels of Testosterone and Estradiol in Independently Living Men. *J. Clin. Endocrinol. Metab.* **2005**, *90*, 157–162. [CrossRef] [PubMed]
14. Global Strategy for Asthma Management and Prevention. Available online: www.ginasthma.org (accessed on 16 February 2020).

15. Heinzerling, L.; Mari, A.; Bergmann, K.C.; Bresciani, M.; Burbach, G.; Darsow, U.; Durham, S.; Fokkens, W.; Gjomarkaj, M.; Haahtela, T.; et al. The skin prick test—European standards. *Clin. Transl. Allergy* **2013**, *3*, 3. [CrossRef]
16. Miller, M.R.; Hankinson, J.A.; Brusasco, V.; Burgos, F.; Casaburi, R.; Coates, A.; Crapo, R.; Enright, P.; Van Der Grinten, C.P.; Gustafsson, P.; et al. Standardisation of spirometry. *Eur. Respir. J.* **2005**, *26*, 319–338. [CrossRef]
17. Wanger, J.; Clausen, J.L.; Coates, A.; Pedersen, O.F.; Brusasco, V.; Burgos, F.; Casaburi, R.; Crapo, R.; Enright, P.; Van Der Grinten, C.P.; et al. Standardisation of the measurement of lung volumes. *Eur. Respir. J.* **2005**, *26*, 511–522. [CrossRef] [PubMed]
18. American Thoracic Society; European Respiratory Society. ATS/ERS recommendations for standardized procedures for the online and offline measurement of exhaled lower respiratory nitric oxide and nasal nitric oxide, 2005. *Am. J. Respir. Crit. Care Med.* **2005**, *171*, 912–930. [CrossRef] [PubMed]
19. Toungoussova, O.; Migliori, G.B.; Barbaro, M.P.; Esposito, L.M.; Dragonieri, S.; Carpagnano, G.E.; Salerno, F.G.; Neri, M.; Spanevello, A. Changes in sputum composition during 15 min of sputum induction in healthy subjects and patients with asthma and chronic obstructive pulmonary disease. *Respir. Med.* **2007**, *101*, 1543–1548. [CrossRef]
20. Assaggaf, H.; Felty, Q. Gender, Estrogen, and Obliterative Lesions in the Lung. *Int. J. Endocrinol.* **2017**, *2017*, 8475701. [CrossRef]
21. Fuentes, N.; Silveyra, P. Endocrine regulation of lung disease and inflammation. *Exp. Biol. Med. (Maywood)* **2018**, *243*, 1313–1322. [CrossRef] [PubMed]
22. Della Torre, F.; Cassani, L.; Segale, M. Asma ed orticaria nell'anziano: Ruolo degli ormoni ipofiso-gonadici in menopausa. *Rass. Geriatr.* **1988**, *24*, 165–171.
23. Jiang, Y.; Zhou, Z.; Ji, Y. Experimental immunology Effects of the recombinant allergen rDer f 2 on neuro-endocrino-immune network in asthmatic mice. *Cent. Eur. J. Immunol.* **2014**, *3*, 294–298. [CrossRef]
24. Mendel, C.M. The free hormone hypothesis. Distinction from the free hormone transport hypothesis. *J. Androl.* **1992**, *13*, 107–116.
25. Bhowmik, A.; Seemungal, T.A.R.; Sapsford, R.J.; Devalia, J.L.; Wedzicha, J.A. Comparison of spontaneous and induced sputum for investigation of airway inflammation in chronic obstructive pulmonary disease. *Thorax* **1998**, *53*, 953–956. [CrossRef]
26. Newcomb, D.C.; Peebles, R.S. Th17-mediated inflammation in asthma. *Curr. Opin. Immunol.* **2013**, *25*, 755–760. [CrossRef]
27. Miyagi, M.; Aoyama, H.; Morishita, M.; Iwamoto, Y. Effects of Sex Hormones on Chemotaxis of Human Peripheral Polymorphonuclear Leukocytes and Monocytes. *J. Periodontol.* **1992**, *63*, 28–32. [CrossRef] [PubMed]
28. Itagaki, T.; Shimizu, I.; Cheng, X.; Yuan, Y.; Oshio, A.; Tamaki, K.; Fukuno, H.; Honda, H.; Okamura, Y.; Ito, S. Opposing effects of oestradiol and progesterone on intracellular pathways and activation processes in the oxidative stress induced activation of cultured rat hepatic stellate cells. *Gut* **2005**, *54*, 1782–1789. [CrossRef] [PubMed]
29. Marin, D.P.; Bolin, A.P.; de Cassia Macedo dos Santos, R.; Curi, R.; Otton, R. Testosterone suppresses oxidative stress in human neutrophils. *Cell Biochem. Funct.* **2010**, *28*, 394–402. [CrossRef] [PubMed]
30. Cutolo, M.; Sulli, A.; Capellino, S.; Villaggio, B.; Montagna, P.; Seriolo, B.; Straub, R.H. Sex hormones influence on the immune system: Basic and clinical aspects in autoimmunity. *Lupus* **2004**, *13*, 635–638. [CrossRef] [PubMed]
31. Abraham, B.; Antó, J.M.; Barreiro, E.; Bel, E.H.; Bonsignore, G.; Bousquet, J.; Castellsague, J.; Chanez, P.; Cibella, F.; Cuttitta, G.; et al. The ENFUMOSA cross-sectional European multicentre study of the clinical phenotype of chronic severe asthma. *Eur. Respir. J.* **2003**, *22*, 470–477. [CrossRef]
32. Moore, W.C.; Meyers, D.A.; Wenzel, S.E.; Teague, W.G.; Li, H.; Li, X.; D'Agostino, R., Jr.; Castro, M.; Curran-Everett, D.; Fitzpatrick, A.M.; et al. Identification of asthma phenotypes using cluster analysis in the severe asthma research program. *Am. J. Respir. Crit. Care Med.* **2010**, *181*, 315–323. [CrossRef] [PubMed]
33. Quek, Y.W.; Sun, H.L.; Ng, Y.Y.; Lee, H.S.; Yang, S.F.; Ku, M.S.; Lu, K.H.; Sheu, J.N.; Lue, K.H. Associations of Serum Leptin with Atopic Asthma and Allergic Rhinitis in Children. *Am. J. Rhinol. Allergy* **2010**, *24*, 354–358. [CrossRef] [PubMed]

34. Beuther, D.A.; Sutherland, E.R. Overweight, obesity, and incident asthma: A meta-analysis of prospective epidemiologic studies. *Am. J. Respir. Crit. Care Med.* **2007**, *175*, 661–666. [CrossRef] [PubMed]
35. Ma, J.; Xiao, L. Association of general and central obesity and atopic and nonatopic asthma in US adults. *J. Asthma* **2013**, *50*, 395–402. [CrossRef] [PubMed]

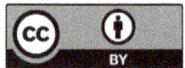
© 2020 by the authors. Licensee MDPI, Basel, Switzerland. This article is an open access article distributed under the terms and conditions of the Creative Commons Attribution (CC BY) license (http://creativecommons.org/licenses/by/4.0/).

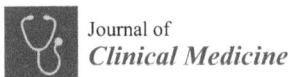

Review

Effective Asthma Management: Is It Time to Let the AIR out of SABA?

Alan Kaplan [1,*], Patrick D. Mitchell [2], Andrew J. Cave [3], Remi Gagnon [4], Vanessa Foran [5] and Anne K. Ellis [6]

1. Family Physician Airways Group of Canada, Edmonton, AB T5X 4P8, Canada
2. Cumming School of Medicine, University of Calgary, Calgary, AB T2N 1N4, Canada; Patrick.Mitchell2@albertahealthservices.ca
3. Department of Family Medicine, Faculty of Medicine and Dentistry, University of Alberta, Edmonton, AB T6G 2R7, Canada; acave@ualberta.ca
4. Association of Allergists and Immunologists of Québec, Montréal, QC H5B 1G8, Canada; rgagnon@csacqc.ca
5. Asthma Canada, Toronto, ON M4S 2Z2, Canada; vanessa.foran@asthma.ca
6. Division of Allergy & Immunology, Department of Medicine, Queen's University, Kingston, ON K7L 3N6, Canada; Anne.Ellis@kingstonhsc.ca
* Correspondence: for4kids@gmail.com

Received: 10 March 2020; Accepted: 21 March 2020; Published: 27 March 2020

Abstract: For years, standard asthma treatment has included short acting beta agonists (SABA), including as monotherapy in patients with mild asthma symptoms. In the Global Initiative for Asthma 2019 strategy for the management of asthma, the authors recommended a significant departure from the traditional treatments. Short acting beta agonists (SABAs) are no longer recommended as the preferred reliever for patients when they are symptomatic and should not be used at all as monotherapy because of significant safety concerns and poor outcomes. Instead, the more appropriate course is the use of a combined inhaled corticosteroid–fast acting beta agonist as a reliever. This paper discusses the issues associated with the use of SABA, the reasons that patients over-use SABA, difficulties that can be expected in overcoming SABA over-reliance in patients, and our evolving understanding of the use of "anti-inflammatory relievers" in our patients with asthma.

Keywords: SABA overuse; systemic steroid overuse; asthma control; mild asthma; ICS adherence; treatment; exacerbation

---

1. Introduction

In 2019, the Global Initiate for Asthma (GINA) changed their strategy for the management of step 1 and step 2 (mild) asthma: Short acting beta agonists (SABAs) as a monotherapy should not be used in patients with mild asthma; rather, patients should be prescribed a combination inhaled corticoid steroid (ICS)–fast acting reliever instead [1]. This change was made because of the recognition that SABA overuse and subsequent ICS underuse are responsible for safety concerns and poor outcomes, including hospitalization and possibly death. This change mostly impacts primary care physicians as they are most frequently providing care for these patients with mild asthma.

The Problem

For many years, the standard asthma treatment has included the use of SABAs, either alone or as part of a therapy including inhaled corticoid steroids (ICSs), to provide rapid relief of symptoms in patients at the time when they are symptomatic, with the administration of oral corticosteroids (OCSs) to manage patients during moderate or severe acute exacerbations. However, with recent evolution in our understanding of the impacts of this reliance of SABA use on patient outcomes, the central role that these agents play in the treatment of asthma has been drawn into question.

While the use of as needed (PRN) SABA provides rapid relief of asthma symptoms, it does not address the underlying inflammatory process and does not protect the patient from exacerbations [2]. Patients that are treated with SABA alone are at higher risk for asthma related death [3] and urgent asthma-related healthcare [4] even if they have good symptom control [5]. Asthma patients treated with SABA monotherapy also have worse long-term outcomes and lower lung function than patients that are treated with low dose maintenance ICSs from the time of diagnosis [6]. Differences between patient and physician views of control and poor communication between patients and physicians about asthma status have been cited as a paradox of asthma management contributing to over-reliance on SABAs and underuse of ICSs [7].

All patients with asthma are at risk of exacerbation, regardless of the severity of the underlying disease [1]. Risk factors or indicators for exacerbation include high SABA use, environmental exposures (smoke, air pollution, or allergens), history of exacerbation, and poor adherence to therapy [1]. The rate of exacerbation is not trivial, even for patients with mild asthma. Clinical trial data show that patients with mild asthma treated with PRN SABAs still have a greater than 20% risk of a moderate to severe exacerbation over the course of one year [8]. In 2011, asthma was the leading cause for hospitalization in Canada, with emergency rooms dealing with more than 64,000 asthma related events [9]. Almost one third of asthma patients have reported having at least one emergency department visit each year [10]. The costs to society are profound; estimates of the direct costs to the health system (including hospitals, drugs, and physician fees) are $1.35 billion for 2020 with indirect costs (long term disability and mortality) adding a further $1.7 billion, for a total of over $3 billion [11]. Costs are expected to rise to $4.2 billion in the next decade [11].

Patients who are treated with SABA monotherapy have a greater risk of severe exacerbation than patients treated with ICSs; these exacerbations are routinely managed through the use of OCSs, typically in short courses or bursts [12]. However, there are very real concerns associated with the prescription of OCSs, particularly with adverse effects of these agents. These effects include increased risk of herpes zoster, cardiovascular events, type 2 diabetes, bone related conditions and fractures, cataracts, obesity, and hypertension [9,13]. The risk is strongly associated with cumulative OCS dose, rather than the maximum dose from a single course. Patients who receive even one to three prescriptions in a year have a 4% increased risk for adverse effects, while patients receiving four or more have a 29% increased risk [13]. However, the risk does not appear to return to baseline; patients who received four or more OCS prescriptions for any 3 years in the prior 10 had a 1.73-fold greater risk for adverse effects than patients who did not receive OCS prescription [13].

There are significant costs associated with OCS exposure to patients with asthma. Comparing patients that have been treated with OCSs to matched OCS untreated patients, long term adverse and costly outcomes have been associated with OCS initiation and have a dosage–response relationship with OCS exposure [14]. Voorham and colleagues found there were profound OCS dose-dependent health-care utilization increases in both general practitioner visits and prescriptions, as well as increases in costs of hospitalizations and general practitioner visits associated with OCS use. A recent Swedish observational study found that asthma patients who were regularly treated with OCSs had triple the health care utilization costs when compared with patients who were not treated with OCSs [15]. The major cost drivers were different in the two groups; the primary cost for OCS non-treated patients were primary care consultations, while the primary costs for OCS users were associated with inpatient care. More than 60% of the total costs for asthma and comorbidities was borne by patients regularly treated with OCSs, with more than 70% of the costs of each of asthma, osteoporosis, and pneumonia resulting from treatment of regular OCS users.

Table 1 illustrates the costs of OCS use in a UK cohort of asthma patients with a range of OCS dose levels [14]. The study noted that the negative impact of OCSs was dose related such that patients with higher calculated doses of ICSs experienced the greatest negative impacts for healthcare utilization, costs, and adverse effects [14].

Table 1. Healthcare resource utilization and costs associated with oral corticosteroid (OCS) use in a matched historical cohort extracted from the UK Clinical Practice Research Datalink Database from 1994 to 2015.

	Annualized Health Care Utilization	
Factor	Non-OCS user IRR[1] (n = 9413)	OCS user IRR[1] (n = 9413)
General Practitioner visits	1.00	1.22
Specialist visits	1.00	1.12
Hospitalization	1.00	1.14
Emergency Department Visits	1.00	1.26
Primary Care Prescriptions	1.00	1.35
	All Cause Health Care Costs	
Year	Non-OCS user Relative Cost	OCS User Relative Cost
Year 1	100%	107%
Year 5	100%	150%
Year 10	100%	170%
Year 15	100%	210%
	15 Year Cumulative Incidence of Adverse Effects	
Adverse Effect	Non-OCS user Incidence (n = 9413)	OCS user Incidence (n = 9413)
Renal Impairment	12.5%	27.9%
Type 2 Diabetes	5.6%	9.5%
Pneumonia	3.5%	11.3%
Cataracts	4.4%	11.0%
Cerebrovascular Event	5.1%	10.0%
Cardio-Cerebrovascular Disease	3.6%	9.9%
Osteoporosis	2.0%	8.0%
Myocardial Infarction	2.8%	7.3%
Heart failure	1.1%	3.6%
Glaucoma	1.7%	3.4%

[1] IRR: incidence rate ratio.

2. Asthma Control

Guidelines recommend reviewing asthma control based on symptoms, in part on the amount of SABAs used per week. The current (2019) GINA strategy recommends SABA use < 3 times per week, with assessment for patients who consume three or more canisters per year (equivalent to 12 puffs per week) as there is an increased risk of asthma attack or exacerbation for patients using three or more canisters per year [1]. However, practicing doctors know that the patient reality is different. Patients value their rescue inhaler (SABA) and use it as needed, often underusing their controller medication (ICS and others).

Poor adherence is a common theme when treating chronic conditions and one that may seem to many health-care practitioners as particularly troubling with asthma. Indeed, poor adherence is common with adherence rates of around 50% in children and 30%–70% in adults (depending on the age, sex, ethnicity, and country) [16]. However, good adherence is associated with fewer exacerbations and better outcomes. The most common pattern is for patients to use medication when they have symptoms and avoid use when symptoms are not present. When symptoms occur, patients will increase their use of SABAs but not their controller medication [17]. Paradoxes of asthma treatment support patients' poor understanding of disease control and support over-reliance on SABA medication [7]. Patients are initially treated with SABA monotherapy when they have infrequent symptoms, so they believe the symptom relief is the goal of therapy, rather than management of the underlying pathophysiology.

They believe that they have the autonomy to make the decision when to use the inhaler. However, as the disease advances, patients lose the autonomy of the decision when to treat (with maintenance controller) and are told to avoid the medication that meets their goals for treatment (the reliever), leading to conflict in their minds [7]. A combination of reliever with anti-inflammatory would then meet both the goals of the clinician and the patient [18].

Practical issues with current guidelines for the treatment of asthma are experienced daily by both physician and patient and limit the effective treatment of this disease. Many of the real issues identified in current practice stem from the series of paradoxes that stem from guideline recommendations for asthma treatment [7,18]. These paradoxes include the following:

- conflicting messaging about the use of SABAs (encouraged in mild asthma but discouraged in more severe disease);
- assuming patient acceptance of advice to avoid use of SABAs, the medication that they perceive provides greatest benefit;
- different safety messages between SABAs and long acting beta-agonists (LABAs), where SABAs are considered safe;
- patient-physican dis-concordance between asthma control and frequency, impact, or severity of their symptoms;
- the patient's perception of loss of autonomy over treatment when switching from a PRN SABA (in step one) to physician prescribed daily controller medication in step two [7].

Further, we now know that regular SABA use increases hyper-responsiveness in the lung, leading to greater sensitivity to triggers [18]. The use of a combination ICS with reliever (either SABA or fast acting LABA) across all patients has a better safety profile and efficacy in reducing exacerbation risk than a SABA alone [7,8,18,19].

3. How Did We Get Here?

With a greater understanding of the importance of reducing asthma exacerbations and the subsequent future risk of asthma-related mortalities, the recommendations for SABA use are being reconsidered. Specifically, for safety reasons, GINA no longer recommends SABA-only treatment in asthma but recommends that patients using three or more canisters of SABA per year should be assessed due to the associated increased future risk for exacerbations, hospitalization, or mortality [1]. A variety of factors increase the risk of exacerbations; patients may be at risk despite asthma severity, disease symptom control, or treatment adherence [20–22].

Historically we can look back to data from New Zealand where there was an epidemic of asthma deaths in the 1980s due to regular use of the extra-potent SABA fenoterol [23]. Further Canadian data from the early 1990s showed that there was a direct correlation between the number of SABA inhalers used and increasing mortality; for every one SABA inhaler increase, the death rate increased by a factor of two [24]. Several epidemiological studies have all reached the same conclusion: (over) reliance on SABA therapy is associated with increased adverse health outcomes including intubation and death [24,25].

Pathophysiologically, we now understand the anti-inflammatory benefit of inhaled corticosteroids (ICSs) on oedema and mucus over the sole acute bronchodilatory effect of SABAs. Previous consensus driven international strategies have recommended SABAs as first-line therapy to relieve immediate asthma symptoms (Figure 1A) [26]. This is despite the fact that asthma is most often characterized as an inflammatory condition characterized by exacerbations and persistent airflow limitations [7,18]. SABAs will resolve the immediate bronchospasm of an allergic trigger but have no inherent anti-inflammatory pharmacological properties and no effect on the late phase reaction. Further, regular use of SABAs have been shown to worsen the delayed inflammatory phase response [27], causing increased bronchial hyper-responsiveness on subsequent exposure to the trigger. Recurrent exposure of the airways to SABAs also contribute to a decreased response to SABA therapy as a reliever [28]. This could explain why regular use of SABAs (≥3 canisters of SABA/year) have an overall detrimental impact on the patient and have been linked to increased OCS use, increased emergency department visits, hospitalization, and disease progression [2,29].

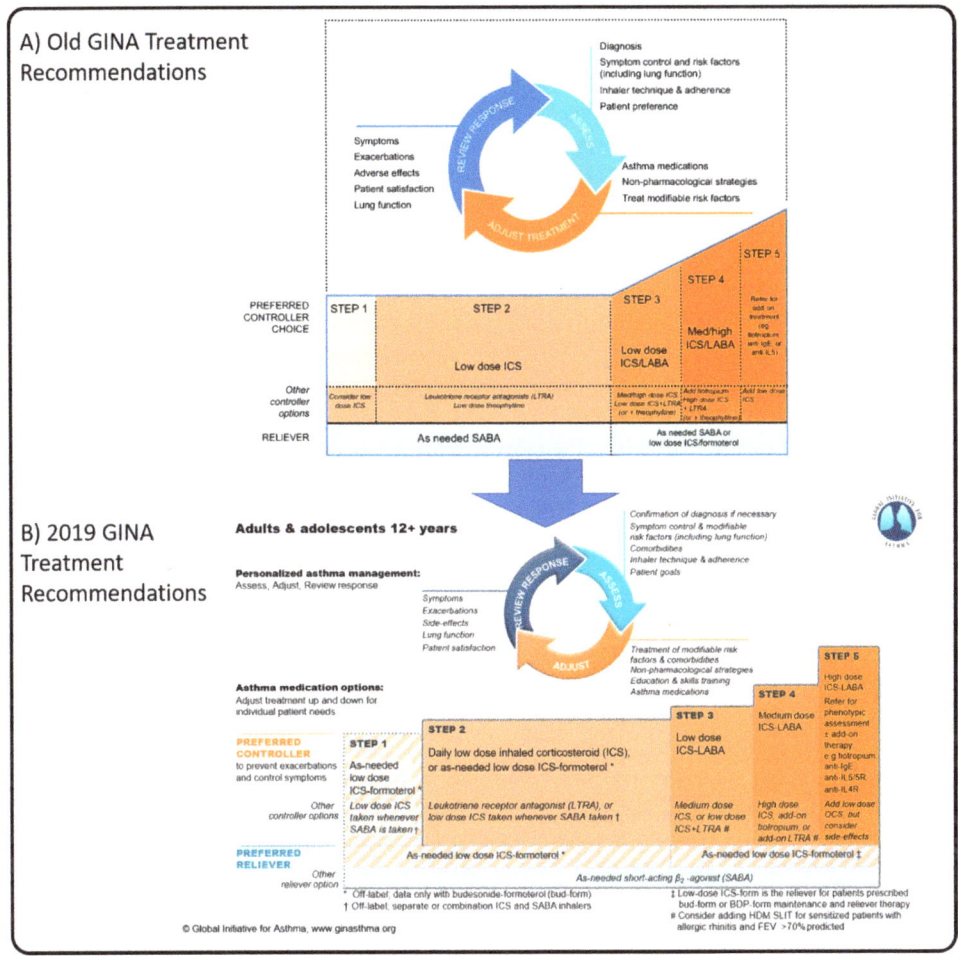

Figure 1. Personalized management for adults and adolescents from the Global Initiative for Asthma Global Strategy for Asthma Management and Prevention for 2018 (**A**) and 2019 (**B**), illustrating the changes to the recommended management in the newest strategy. Adapted from GINA 2018 [26] and GINA 2019 [1]. BDP: beclomethasone dipropionate; FEV: forced expiratory volume; HDM: house dust mite; LTRA: Leukotriene Receptor Antagonist; SLIT, sub-lingual therapy.

The risk of SABA over-reliance has been clearly identified in a series of case reviews and studies. In a review of 192 patients in the UK who died from asthma in 2012, it was clear that there was a significant over-reliance on SABAs with 39% of those patients receiving 12 SABA inhalers per year, and 4% receiving 50 SABA inhalers in one year [30]! In contrast, the use of controllers was low, with 80% receiving less than the optimal 12 prescriptions per year and 38% receiving less than four per year. Another study of over 35,000 UK patients with asthma showed a direct relationship between the frequency of SABAs prescribed beyond the baseline of 1–3 per year and risk of hospital admission for asthma. The author's conclusion was that there is a progressive risk of hospital admission associated with the prescription of 3 or more canisters of SABA per year [31].

A qualitative study [32] examined the reasons for SABA over-reliance in young adults with asthma. Reasons given for SABA inhaler over-reliance included wanting a short-term quick fix for asthma symptoms, cost, poor adaptation to illness, reducing stigma of having a chronic illness, asthma having career and social issues, fear of symptoms, anger at having illness, feeling that they cannot survive without it (the blue one), but that they could survive without the maintenance medicine. These issues require disease education and reinforcement of best practices.

It has been shown that shared decision making between the patient and clinician improves adherence to asthma therapy [33]. However, it did require four additional steps: i) identifying patient goals and preferences; ii) summarizing patient goals and preferences; iii) discussing relative merits of different treatment options in relation to goals and preferences; and iv) negotiating a decision about a treatment regimen. One study found that after one year, there was an increased total days' controller prescription by an average of 77 days and by 9.6 ICS canister equivalents, increased quality of life by 0.4 points out of 5, reduced unscheduled asthma physician visits, reduced SABA acquisition by 1.6 canister equivalents, and doubling of the likelihood of having well controlled asthma [33].

4. Solutions

Data has shown that simultaneous anti-inflammatory and reliever use [8,34–36] demonstrates similar outcomes in asthma control with significantly reduced exacerbation rates over SABA alone. This has led to a paradigm shift which has been reflected in a change in the GINA strategy. As of 2019, based on strong evidence that SABA-only treatment increases the risk of severe exacerbations and asthma related death, SABA therapy should no longer be considered for monotherapy in asthma, with anti-inflammatory reliever therapy now the preferred reliever in adults (Figure 1B). Further, the recommendation in children is now the co-administration of ICSs with SABAs to ensure inflammation treatment is optimized at the time it is needed [1].

This change was based on significant evidence that SABA-only treatment increases the risk of severe exacerbations and asthma-related death and the supporting data that adding ICSs significantly reduces the risk. A large body of evidence from randomized controlled trials and observational studies shows that low dose ICSs substantially reduce the risk of severe exacerbations, hospitalizations, and death [3,4,37,38]. One study demonstrated that regular low dose ICS reduces the risk of asthma exacerbations by 60% and improves asthma control days by half [37]. Further, more recent data [8,34] has demonstrated that treatment with budesonide-formoterol (ICS-long-acting β-agonist) solely as-needed prevented exacerbations and loss of lung function, however, was less effective at mitigating symptoms than regular ICS maintenance therapy. Unfortunately, many patients do not adhere with regular ICS therapy and are not availing themselves of this protection. Patients require ICS at the time of worsening symptoms but have learned that SABAs provide the benefits of immediate relief that they seek [7]. Coupling the delivery of ICSs with a reliever makes use of the patient goals for therapy (i.e., fast relief) to ensure that the required anti-inflammatory is delivered when it is most needed, at the time of the asthma worsening [38].

The GINA strategy notes that patients receive either symptom-driven (in mild asthma) or daily ICS-containing controller treatment to reduce the risk of severe exacerbations and asthma-related death. Further recommendations are for as-needed controller treatment in mild asthma, with a preferred controller being low dose ICS–formoterol taken as needed for relief of symptoms and before exercise [1]. Currently, only budesonide–formoterol has been studied in Canada in this role; beclomethasone–formoterol has been approved in Europe for the treatment of moderate to severe asthma only. The use of SABA reliever in ICS controller therapy (either with or without a LABA) is associated with a higher risk of asthma exacerbation, compared to using budesonide–formoterol as maintenance and reliever, in patients over the age of 12 years [35]. At the time of this writing, only studies investigating budesonide–formoterol in this role have been conducted. Different ICS components may have different safety outcomes, and certainly different LABA compounds could lack the rapid onset required. While this concept may be applicable to other ICS–formoterol products, without controlled trials, recommending other ICS–formoterol products in this role would not be appropriate.

There are a number of questions that remain unanswered for many patients. Most trials of the anti-inflammatory reliever strategy have been performed using budesonide–formoterol in patients that are prescribed budesonide–formoterol as a controller (when they require a controller). However, in practice, some patients are using and are effectively managed with combination products other than budesonide–formoterol (such as fluticasone–salmeterol or mometasone–formoterol). The impact of budesonide–formoterol used as an as-needed reliever in the context of another controller (either a different ICS–LABA or just an ICS alone) has been poorly studied. In this case, patients who are well-controlled on these other controller medications should not be transitioned to the new strategy.

The continued use of a SABA monotherapy rather than an anti-inflammatory reliever may be appropriate in some patients. Patients with non-eosinophilic asthma (including neutrophilic asthma) and patients with true exercise induced bronchospasm (i.e., exercise induced asthma) may not benefit from the steroid component. Further, the Health Canada authorization for budesonide–formoterol indicates the combination as an anti-inflammatory reliever in patients with mild and persistent symptoms. SABAs should also be continued in patients that are using other ICS–LABA combinations as maintenance products; using budesonide–formoterol a reliever may not be appropriate in patients treated with a different ICS–LABA combination as these combinations have not been studied [39]. It is also important to ensure an accurate diagnosis of asthma in the patient; patients with mild COPD (or other ailments that may present as asthma) should not be treated with an ICS.

There may be some perceived disadvantages of anti-inflammatory reliever therapy. The side effects of the combination product are mild, well understood (as budesonide–formoterol is widely used as a maintenance therapy), and are generally related to the ICS component. The strategy encourages a lower total dose of the ICS as the inflammation is only treated at the time it is occurring, preventing overtreatment. Patients may be concerned with the cost of the product (when compared with short acting relievers). However, use of an anti-inflammatory reliever may ultimately reduce the quantity of the product used as well as reducing symptoms, partially negating the cost differential. There may be a concern with the total ICS dose in patients using an anti-inflammatory reliever strategy; however, the total dose for such a strategy will be less than patients using a SABA reliever in studies including mild, moderate, and severe asthma patients.

5. Conclusions

Despite the evidence, SABA over-reliance continues, with decreased ICS use due to poor adherence, increased OCS use due to exacerbations (typically more than 1 event per year for most patients), increased emergency department visits, and hospitalizations for our patients with asthma. While the negative effect of SABA over-reliance is understood, both clinicians and patients continue to reinforce this behaviour. We need to review SABA use with our patients, particularly to identify those using 3 or more SABA inhalers per year. In those patients, clinicians need to work with the patient to educate on the new GINA strategy of symptom-driven (mild asthma) or daily ICS-containing controller treatment, with as-needed controller treatment (low dose ICS–formoterol) taken as needed for relief of symptoms in place of SABA therapy. Data clearly shows that regular use of ICSs is the best strategy. However, lack of adherence to this often precludes use of ICSs. By taking advantage of the patient's own behaviour to use an anti-inflammatory at the time of the reliever, we can impact behaviours and ensure an ICS is used at the time it is needed to control airway inflammation.

Author Contributions: A.K. was the principle author of the manuscript. A.K.E. is the chair of the Asthma Zero group. All authors contributed equally to the content and themes of the manuscript and provided input into the development and content throughout the process of preparing the manuscript. All authors have read and agreed to the published version of the manuscript.

Funding: Financial support for preparation of this manuscript was provided by AstraZeneca Canada Inc.

Acknowledgments: The authors wish to acknowledge the members of the Asthma Zero Steering group for their valuable insights into the creation of this manuscript. The Asthma Zero Steering group members are A.E., S.C., F.D., V.F., D.P., P.G., A.K., A.C., P.M., J.P.D., and R.G.

Conflicts of Interest: The authors declare no conflict of interest. The funders had no role in developing the editorial content of this manuscript. A.K. is a member of an advisory board or speaker's bureau for Astra Zeneca, Boerhringer-Ingelheim, Covis, Griffols, GSK, Pfizer, Purdue, Novartis, NovoNordisk, Sanofi, Talecris, and Trudel. P.D.M. reports receiving consulting fees from A.Z., GSK, Teva, and Sanofi, honorarium payments from A.Z., GSK, Teva, Sanofi, and Novartis, and unrestricted research grant support from A.Z., GSK, and Teva. A.J.C. has received research grants from The Lung Association, Grifols Canada, Alberta Innovates, and AstraZeneca and received honoraria from GSK, AstraZeneca, Sanofi, and Boerhinger-Ingelheim.

References

1. Global Initiative for Asthma. Global Strategy for Asthma Management and Prevention, 2019. 2019. Available online: www.ginasthma.org (accessed on 5 March 2020).
2. Stanford, R.H.; Shah, M.B.; D'Souza, A.O.; Dhamane, A.D.; Schatz, M. Short-acting β-agonist use and its ability to predict future asthma-related outcomes. *Ann. Allergy Asthma Immunol.* **2012**, *109*, 403–407. [CrossRef] [PubMed]
3. Suissa, S.; Ernst, P.; Benayoun, S.; Baltzan, M.; Cai, B. Low-dose inhaled corticosteroids and the prevention of death from asthma. *N. Engl. J. Med.* **2000**, *343*, 332–336. [CrossRef]
4. Suissa, S.; Ernst, P.; Kezouh, A. Regular use of inhaled corticosteroids and the long term prevention of hospitalisation for asthma. *Thorax* **2002**, *57*, 880–884. [CrossRef] [PubMed]
5. Reddel, H.K.; Busse, W.W.; Pedersen, S.; Tan, W.C.; Chen, Y.-Z.; Jorup, C.; Lythgoe, D.; O'Byrne, P.M. Should recommendations about starting inhaled corticosteroid treatment for mild asthma be based on symptom frequency: A post-hoc efficacy analysis of the START study. *Lancet* **2017**, *389*, 157–166. [CrossRef]
6. Haahtela, T.; Järvinen, M.; Kava, T.; Kiviranta, K.; Koskinen, S.; Lehtonen, K.; Nikander, K.; Persson, T.; Reinikainen, K.; Selroos, O.; et al. Comparison of a beta 2-agonist, terbutaline, with an inhaled corticosteroid, budesonide, in newly detected asthma. *N. Engl. J. Med.* **1991**, *325*, 388–392. [CrossRef] [PubMed]
7. O'Byrne, P.M.; Jenkins, C.; Bateman, E.D. The paradoxes of asthma management: Time for a new approach? *Eur. Respir. J.* **2017**, *50*. [CrossRef]
8. O'Byrne, P.M.; FitzGerald, J.M.; Bateman, E.D.; Barnes, P.J.; Zhong, N.; Keen, C.; Jorup, C.; Lamarca, R.; Ivanov, S.; Reddel, H.K. Inhaled Combined Budesonide–Formoterol as Needed in Mild Asthma. *N. Engl. J. Med.* **2018**. [CrossRef]
9. Asthma Society of Canada. Severe Asthma: The Canadian Patient Journey. 2014. Available online: https://www.asthma.ca/wp-content/uploads/2017/06/SAstudy.pdf (accessed on 28 September 2018).
10. Rowe, B.H.; Villa-Roel, C.; Abu-Laban, R.B.; Stenstrom, R.; Mackey, D.; Stiell, I.; Campbell, S.; Young, B. Admissions to Canadian hospitals for acute asthma: A prospective, multicentre study. *Can. Respir. J.* **2010**, *17*, 25–30. [CrossRef]
11. The Conference Board of Canada, Louis Theriault, Gregory Hermus, Danielle Goldfarb, Carole Stonebridge, Fares Bounajm. Cost Risk Analysis for Chronic Lung Disease in Canada. Available online: https://www.conferenceboard.ca/e-library/abstract.aspx?did=4585 (accessed on 11 September 2019).
12. Chapman, K.R.; Verbeek, P.R.; White, J.G.; Rebuck, A.S. Effect of a short course of prednisone in the prevention of early relapse after the emergency room treatment of acute asthma. *N. Engl. J. Med.* **1991**, *324*, 788–794. [CrossRef]
13. Sadatsafavi, M.; Rousseau, R.; Chen, W.; Zhang, W.; Lynd, L.; FitzGerald, J.M. The preventable burden of productivity loss due to suboptimal asthma control: A population-based study. *Chest* **2014**, *145*, 787–793. [CrossRef]
14. Voorham, J.; Xu, X.; Price, D.B.; Golam, S.; Davis, J.; Ling, J.Z.J.; Kerkhof, M.; Ow, M.; Tran, T.N. Healthcare resource utilization and costs associated with incremental systemic corticosteroid exposure in asthma. *Allergy* **2019**, *74*, 273–283. [CrossRef]
15. Janson, C.; Lisspers, K.; Ställberg, B.; Johansson, G.; Telg, G.; Thuresson, M.; Christensen, H.N.; Larsson, K. Health care resource utilization and cost for asthma patients regularly treated with oral corticosteroids—A Swedish observational cohort study (PACEHR). *Respir. Res.* **2018**, *19*, 168. [CrossRef]

16. Engelkes, M.; Janssens, H.M.; Jongste, J.C.; de Sturkenboom, M.C.J.M.; Verhamme, K.M.C. Medication adherence and the risk of severe asthma exacerbations: A systematic review. *Eur. Respir. J.* **2015**, *45*, 396–407. [CrossRef]
17. Partridge, M.R.; van der Molen, T.; Myrseth, S.-E.; Busse, W.W. Attitudes and actions of asthma patients on regular maintenance therapy: The INSPIRE study. *BMC Pulm. Med.* **2006**, *6*, 13. [CrossRef]
18. Beasley, R.; Bird, G.; Harper, J.; Weatherall, M. The further paradoxes of asthma management: Time for a new approach across the spectrum of asthma severity. *Eur. Respir. J.* **2018**, *52*. [CrossRef] [PubMed]
19. Papi, A.; Canonica, G.W.; Maestrelli, P.; Paggiaro, P.; Olivieri, D.; Pozzi, E.; Crimi, N.; Vignola, A.M.; Morelli, P.; Nicolini, G.; et al. Rescue use of beclomethasone and albuterol in a single inhaler for mild asthma. *N. Engl. J. Med.* **2007**, *356*, 2040–2052. [CrossRef] [PubMed]
20. Papi, A.; Ryan, D.; Soriano, J.B.; Chrystyn, H.; Bjermer, L.; Rodriguez-Roisin, R.; Dolovich, M.B.; Harris, M.; Wood, L.; Batsiou, M.; et al. Relationship of Inhaled Corticosteroid Adherence to Asthma Exacerbations in Patients with Moderate-to-Severe Asthma. *J. Allergy Clin. Immunol. Pract.* **2018**, *6*, 1989–1998.e3. [CrossRef] [PubMed]
21. Price, D.; Fletcher, M.; van der Molen, T. Asthma control and management in 8,000 European patients: The REcognise Asthma and LInk to Symptoms and Experience (REALISE) survey. *NPJ Prim. Care Respir. Med.* **2014**, *24*, 14009. [CrossRef]
22. Kang, H.-R.; Song, H.J.; Nam, J.H.; Hong, S.-H.; Yang, S.-Y.; Ju, S.; Lee, S.W.; Kim, T.-B.; Kim, H.-L.; Lee, E.-K. Risk factors of asthma exacerbation based on asthma severity: A nationwide population-based observational study in South Korea. *BMJ Open* **2018**, *8*, e020825. [CrossRef]
23. Crane, J.; Flatt, A.; Jackson, R.; Ball, M.; Pearce, N.; Burgess, C.; Kwong, T.; Beasley, R. Prescribed fenoterol and death from asthma in New Zealand, 1981–1983: Case-control study. *Lancet* **1989**, *1*, 917–922. [CrossRef]
24. Spitzer, W.O.; Suissa, S.; Ernst, P.; Horwitz, R.I.; Habbick, B.; Cockcroft, D.; Boivin, J.-F.; McNutt, M.; Buist, A.S.; Rebuck, A.S. The use of beta-agonists and the risk of death and near death from asthma. *N. Engl. J. Med.* **1992**, *326*, 501–506. [CrossRef] [PubMed]
25. Fitzgerald, J.M.; Lemiere, C.; Lougheed, M.D.; Ducharme, F.M.; Dell, S.D.; Ramsey, C.; Yang, C.; Côté, A.; Watson, W.; Olivenstein, R.; et al. Recognition and management of severe asthma: A Canadian Thoracic Society position statement. *Can. J. Respir. Crit. Care, Sleep Med.* **2017**, *1*, 199–221. [CrossRef]
26. Global Initiative for Asthma. Global Strategy for Asthma Management and Prevention, 2018. 2018. Available online: www.ginasthma.org (accessed on 11 May 2018).
27. Gauvreau, G.M.; Jordana, M.; Watson, R.M.; Cockroft, D.W.; O'Byrne, P.M. Effect of regular inhaled albuterol on allergen-induced late responses and sputum eosinophils in asthmatic subjects. *Am. J. Respir. Crit. Care Med.* **1997**, *156*, 1738–1745. [CrossRef] [PubMed]
28. Lohse, M.J.; Benovic, J.L.; Caron, M.G.; Lefkowitz, R.J. Multiple pathways of rapid beta 2-adrenergic receptor desensitization. Delineation with specific inhibitors. *J. Biol. Chem.* **1990**, *265*, 3202–3211. [PubMed]
29. Chen, W.; FitzGerald, J.M.; Lynd, L.D.; Sin, D.D.; Sadatsafavi, M. Long-Term Trajectories of Mild Asthma in Adulthood and Risk Factors of Progression. *J. Allergy Clin. Immunol. Pract.* **2018**, *6*, 2024–2032.e5. [CrossRef]
30. Royal College of Physicians. Why Asthma Still Kills. RCP London. Available online: https://www.rcplondon.ac.uk/projects/outputs/why-asthma-still-kills (accessed on 19 July 2019).
31. Hull, S.A.; McKibben, S.; Homer, K.; Taylor, S.J.; Pike, K.; Griffiths, C. Asthma prescribing, ethnicity and risk of hospital admission: An analysis of 35,864 linked primary and secondary care records in East London. *NPJ Prim. Care Respir. Med.* **2016**, *26*, 16049. [CrossRef]
32. Cole, S.; Seale, C.; Griffiths, C. "The blue one takes a battering" why do young adults with asthma overuse bronchodilator inhalers? A qualitative study. *BMJ Open* **2013**, *3*. [CrossRef]
33. Wilson, S.R.; Strub, P.; Buist, A.S.; Knowles, S.B.; Lavori, P.W.; Lapidus, J.; Vollmer, W.M. Shared treatment decision making improves adherence and outcomes in poorly controlled asthma. *Am. J. Respir. Crit. Care Med.* **2010**, *181*, 566–577. [CrossRef]
34. Bateman, E.D.; Reddel, H.K.; O'Byrne, P.M.; Barnes, P.J.; Zhong, N.; Keen, C.; Jorup, C.; Lamarca, R.; Siwek-Posluszna, A.; Fitzgerald, J.M. As-Needed Budesonide-Formoterol versus Maintenance Budesonide in Mild Asthma. *N. Engl. J. Med.* **2018**, *378*, 1877–1887. [CrossRef]

35. Sobieraj, D.M.; Weeda, E.R.; Nguyen, E.; Coleman, C.I.; White, C.M.; Lazarus, S.C.; Blake, K.V.; Lang, J.E.; Baker, W.L. Association of Inhaled Corticosteroids and Long-Acting β-Agonists as Controller and Quick Relief Therapy with Exacerbations and Symptom Control in Persistent Asthma: A Systematic Review and Meta-analysis. *JAMA* **2018**, *319*, 1485–1496. [CrossRef]
36. Beasley, R.; Holliday, M.; Reddel, H.K.; Braithwaite, I.; Ebmeier, S.; Hancox, R.J.; Harrison, T.; Houghton, C.; Oldfield, K.; Papi, A.; et al. Controlled Trial of Budesonide-Formoterol as Needed for Mild Asthma. *N. Engl. J. Med.* **2019**, *380*, 2020–2030. [CrossRef] [PubMed]
37. O'Byrne, P.M.; Barnes, P.J.; Rodríguez-Roisin, R.; Runnerstrom, E.; Sandstrom, T.; Svensson, K.; Tattersfield, A. Low dose inhaled budesonide and formoterol in mild persistent asthma: The OPTIMA randomized trial. *Am. J. Respir. Crit. Care Med.* **2001**, *164 Pt 1*, 1392–1397. [CrossRef]
38. Pauwels, R.A.; Pedersen, S.; Busse, W.W.; Tan, W.C.; Chen, Y.-Z.; Ohlsson, S.V.; Ullman, A.; Lamm, C.J.; O'Byrne, P.M. Early intervention with budesonide in mild persistent asthma: A randomised, double-blind trial. *Lancet* **2003**, *361*, 1071–1076. [CrossRef]
39. Licskai, C.; Yang, C.L.; Lemiere, C.; Ducharme, F.M.; Lougheed, M.D.; Radhakrishnan, D.; Podgers, D.; Ramsey, C.; Samanta, T.; Côté, A.; et al. Are the 2019 Global Initiative for Asthma (GINA) strategy recommendations applicable to the Canadian context? *Can. J. Respir. Crit. Care Sleep Med.* **2019**, *4*, 3–6. [CrossRef]

© 2020 by the authors. Licensee MDPI, Basel, Switzerland. This article is an open access article distributed under the terms and conditions of the Creative Commons Attribution (CC BY) license (http://creativecommons.org/licenses/by/4.0/).

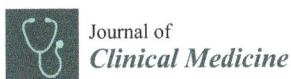

Review

Use of Sublingual Immunotherapy for Aeroallergens in Children with Asthma

Carlo Caffarelli [1],*, Carla Mastrorilli [2], Michela Procaccianti [1] and Angelica Santoro [1]

[1] Clinica Pediatrica, Dipartimento di Medicina e Chirurgia, Università di Parma, Azienda Ospedaliero-Universitaria di Parma, 43126 Parma, Italy; michela.procaccianti@outlook.it (M.P.); angelica.santoro204@gmail.com (A.S.)
[2] UO Pediatria e Pronto Soccorso, Azienda Ospedaliero-Universitaria Consorziale Policlinico, Ospedale Pediatrico Giovanni XXIII, 70126 Bari, Italy; carla.mastrorilli@icloud.com
* Correspondence: carlo.caffarelli@unipr.it; Tel.: +39-521-702207

Received: 30 September 2020; Accepted: 20 October 2020; Published: 21 October 2020

Abstract: Asthma is a heterogeneous disease that in children is often allergen-driven with a type 2 inflammation. Sublingual immunotherapy represents an important progress in the use of personalized medicine in children with allergic asthma. It is a viable option for house dust mite-driven asthma and in subjects with the asthma associated with allergic rhinitis. The use and indications for isolated asthma caused by other allergens are still controversial owing to heterogeneity of commercially available products and methodological limitations of studies in children. Nevertheless, most studies and meta-analyses found the efficacy of sublingual immunotherapy. Sublingual immunotherapy is safe but cannot be recommended in children with uncontrolled asthma.

Keywords: asthma; children; efficacy; house dust mite; pollen allergy; rhinitis; safety; sublingual immunotherapy

1. Introduction

Asthma is a chronic disease affecting 10%–15% of school-aged children [1,2]. First-line treatment for allergic asthma consists of such medicines as inhaled corticosteroids, long-acting beta2-agonists and short-acting beta2-agonists as needed with the aim of minimizing symptoms, improving lung function, and reducing inflammation. Notwithstanding, some children need additional treatment to improve asthma control. Moreover, in patients who achieve control, symptoms can return upon discontinuation of drugs. Different response to the same therapy can be due to a distinctive asthma endotype that indicates a subtype of the disease with a distinct underlying pathophysiological mechanism. In childhood, two forms of asthma have been conventionally studied. The type2 (T2)-high endotype can be allergic [3] or nonallergic and it is characterized by an eosinophilic airway inflammation, while in the T2-low endotype, a neutrophilic or paucigranulocytic airway inflammation is found [4]. Most children have allergic asthma that may be considered a phenotype, with early onset, atopic background, family atopic history, allergic sensitization to common inhaled allergens, eosinophil inflammation, and bronchial hyperreactivity that overlaps with eosinophilic and T2 asthma [5]. In this promising era of precision medicine, matching asthmatic patients with the T2-high endotype allows "personalizing" more effective therapeutic choices that target the airway T2 pathway. They include biologicals and allergen specific immunotherapy (AIT) in asthmatics who partly respond or do not respond to first-line treatment or have a recurrence after a suspension. AIT has been the first attempt of precision medicine and it is tailored to the specific IgE that elicits the reaction. AIT is the only disease-modifying treatment for patients with IgE-mediated allergy due to airborne allergens. It consists of repetitive administration of the allergen extract that provokes symptoms with the purpose of inducing allergen tolerance in allergic asthma by targeting the underlying mechanisms and modifying the immunological response.

Subcutaneous AIT (SCIT) has been the only accepted effective AIT for allergic rhinitis and asthma over several years [6] and it still represents the standard treatment for hymenoptera venom hypersensitivity. SCIT may rarely induce unpredictable anaphylactic reactions. Moreover, children can be annoyed by repeated injections that require visiting a doctor's office. So, alternative safer and more comfortable routes of allergen administration that may allow self-administration at home have been investigated. The first randomized double-blind placebo-controlled trials (RDBPCT) of such routes took place in 1986 and studied sublingual AIT (SLIT) [7]. Subsequently, a remarkable number of clinical studies on SLIT was published showing indirectly an efficacy not far from that of SCIT [8,9] even if head-to-head studies are lacking. SLIT has been quickly recognized in official documents as an alternative to SCIT in respiratory allergy at variance from other routes [10–14]. Furthermore, SLIT has been used for other allergy-driven diseases, such as atopic dermatitis [15]. Both SCIT and SLIT share similar mechanisms, that involve induction of allergen-specific IgG4, stimulation of IgE-blocking IgG antibodies, T-cell tolerance [16]. These mechanisms suppress the specific Th2 immune response and prevent further exacerbations. In SLIT, an important role for antigen tolerance is played by the uptake of the allergen by dendritic cells of oral mucosa [17]. SLIT is specific for the allergen causing IgE-mediated asthma but not for asthma in itself [10]. So, we have analyzed the use of SLIT in asthmatic children, including an approach to its prescription that considers differences between allergens and suggestions for practice.

2. Product-Related Considerations

SLIT vaccines are available as liquid drops or tablets that are swallowed after keeping under the tongue for 1–2 min. Sublingual formulations are not equivalent since they vary according to the manufacturer in the diluent, preservatives, unit of measurement of potency, dosage, and schedules. The diversity in marketed products has led to heterogeneity in the way national regulators deal with different products. In most countries, AIT products usually require a marketing permission like other drugs [18]. However, SLIT products are also commercialized and routinely used in many countries as "named patient products" that just need to be prepared according to the Good Manufacturing Practice to be commercialized.

In the past 15 years, several big trials investigated orodispersible tablets with standardized determination of relevant allergen content of the extracts in RDBPCT involving a large number of children and adults with allergic rhinitis and/or asthma. Those studies characterized the optimal maintenance dose of each product [19]. Furthermore, they allowed for the approval of SLIT tablets for timothy, 5-grass, house dust mites (HDM), trees (birch), ragweed, and Japanese cedar by regulating authorities as medicinal products in several countries. Many SLIT products are marketed as solutions that are administered with a dropper, mini-pumps, or single-dose vials. The optimum dose with liquid extracts remains approximate [20] since trials evaluated a small number of children and they were not designed for registration. The mean number of children with asthma due to HDM in the active arm in 8 RDBPCTs [21–28] was 26 and the cumulative dose that was found to reduce asthma symptoms varied from 249.6 mcg Der P1 [23] to 1700 mcg Der P1 [26].

Regarding allergy to grass, SLIT with higher cumulative doses (4068 IR versus 18,031 IR) was associated with a significant low symptom/medication score [29].

SLIT with a mixed *Betula verrucosa*, *Corylus avellana* and *Alnus glutinosa* extract has a similar efficacy at a cumulative dose of 1.058 mcg (major pollen tree allergens) and of 8820 mcg (major pollen tree allergens) in 61 asthmatic children [30].

Cumulative effective doses for Par j varied from 20.3 mcg [23] to 52.2 mg [31].

At variance from SCIT, in SLIT, the build-up phase with increasing doses usually lasts a few days, or it is unnecessary, and the treatment starts with the maintenance dose. The maintenance dose can be administered according to the manufacturer: once a day, on alternate days, twice weekly [32]. SLIT for seasonal allergens can be discontinued at the beginning of the season (preseasonal treatment), at the end of the season (pre-coseasonal) or administered continuously. SLIT for perennial allergens is usually administered all year-round. A SLIT course of 3 years is recommended to achieve better long-term results [33–35]. However, a prospective study found that a treatment of 4 years slightly improved efficacy and long-term benefits in adults [36].

3. Sublingual Immunotherapy for Asthma

Several systematic reviews and trials have been conducted on the use of SLIT in asthmatic children. Meta-analyses have been hampered by heterogeneity among selected studies in population, allergens, products, outcomes, doses, duration of treatment. It is noteworthy that efficacy and safety should be characterized for each formulation because of differences between sublingual products. Furthermore, meta-analyses have been limited by power of the trials since most of them studied primarily patients with allergic rhinitis [16]. Allergic rhinitis, which affects 60–80% of asthmatic children [37,38], is the most frequent comorbidity and it is associated with worse asthma control. Furthermore, not validated instruments [1,39] were used and asthmatic exacerbations [40] at the time of the studies were not considered as the outcome that the authors should have tried to influence [2]. Even if these shortcomings questioned the conclusions [41], most meta-analyses and systematic reviews [6,42,43] showed the efficacy of SLIT in asthmatic children.

4. House Dust Mites

In asthmatic adolescents and adults, the findings of large studies [44–46] provided evidence of efficacy of HDM SLIT tablets. As a consequence, HDM SLIT has been incorporated in the Global Initiative for Asthma Report (GINA) recommendations [40] as an add-on treatment for HDM allergic asthma in adults with allergic rhinitis who have exacerbations despite a low-medium dose of inhaled corticosteroids if the forced expiratory volume per 1 s (FEV1) is greater than the 70% predicted. Therefore, patients with severe asthma receiving a high dose of inhaled corticosteroids [40] would not be given AIT. However, in the European Academy of Allergy and Clinical Immunology (EAACI) Guidelines [2], HDM SLIT tablets are recommended as an add-on treatment for adults with controlled and partially controlled HDM-driven allergic asthma irrespective of severity of asthma. In RDBPCT that included adolescents and adults, the efficacy of HDM SLIT tablets and drops has been shown [47,48] and they also have spared inhaled corticosteroid [49,50].

In children, ten RDBPTs [21–27,51–53] found that HDM SLIT drops improved asthma symptoms and reduced use of medication (Table 1). The systematic review by Rice et al. [39] found that HDM SLIT improved FEV1. An RDBPCT in a pediatric population reported negative results for HDM SLIT [28]. However, nearly all children had no asthmatic symptoms at the baseline so that lack of benefit could have been anticipated.

5. Grass Pollen

Several reports have shown the efficacy of grass pollen SLIT (Table 1). A large regulatory trial conducted with grass SLIT tablets in children with allergic rhinitis showed a significant improvement in the asthma symptom score but not in the medication use [54], while Rolinck-Werninghaus reported a decrease in the medication score [55]. Stelmach et al. [55] reported that grass SLIT significantly improved asthma symptoms and reduced the medication score in children. Dhami et al. [6] performed a systematic review and a meta-analysis of RDBPCTs on AIT for asthma in children and adults. They found that AIT was effective in decreasing the symptom score both in children and adults and the medication score in children and suggested (but not confirmed) in adults. AIT to grass pollen was effective in reducing the symptom score and the suggested (but not confirmed) medication score. Furthermore, SCIT was effective in reducing respiratory symptoms and drug consumption whereas SLIT was suggested but not confirmed to reduce the symptom and medication scores. However, only one study with SLIT in children [56] was reported [6]. If we look at real life, it has been reported that grass SLIT tablets for allergic rhinitis decrease the number of dispensed prescriptions for asthma medications [57].

6. Trees and Ragweed

Most data on AIT efficacy against tree pollen allergy have been shown in adult studies. A systematic review [42] reported two trials [55,58] showing the effectiveness of SLIT for asthma due to tree pollen allergy in children. A RDBPCT [59] found that SLIT to parietaria significantly reduced nonspecific bronchial hyperresponsiveness to methacholine. Recently, in a RDBPCT, Biedermann et al. [60] found that sublingual tablets containing a standardized birch extract were effective in 634 adolescents or adults with rhinoconjunctivitis caused by birch pollen and in the subpopulation with asthma and reduced the Asthma Control Test score.

Regarding ragweed, a RDBPCT by Nolte et al. [61] showed that ragweed SLIT tablets improved symptoms and medication use in children with rhinoconjunctivitis to ragweed pollen and reduced asthma symptoms and short-acting beta2-agonist use.

Data regarding efficacy of tree and ragweed SLIT in asthmatic children are reported in Table 1.

Table 1. Trials on SLIT efficacy carried out in children with asthma.

Author, Year	Trial	Allergen Extract	Age (Years)	Population (Active/Controls)	AIT Duration (Months)	Outcome
Tari et al., 1990 [21]	RDBPC	HDM	<12	30/28	30	↓ bronchial hyperreactivity
Hirsch et al., 1997 [22]	RDBPC	HDM	6–16	15/15	12	↓ asthma symptoms
Paino et al., 2000 [23]	RDBPC	HDM	8–15	12/12	24	↓ asthma symptoms ↓ medication use
Bahçeciler et al., 2001 [24]	RDBPC	HDM	8–15	7/8	6	↓ asthma attacks ↑ PEF
Ippoliti et al., 2003 [25]	RDBPC	HDM	5–12	47/39	6	↓ asthma symptoms ↓ ECP, IL-13, PRL
Lue et al., 2006 [26]	RDBPC	HDM	6–12	10/10	6	↓ asthma symptoms ↑ IgG4, total IgE ↓ eosinophil count ↑ lung function
Niu et al., 2006 [27]	RDBPC	HDM	6–12	49/48	6	↓ asthma symptoms ↓ lung function
Pham-Thi et al., 2007 [28]	RDBPC	HDM	5–16	55/56	18	↓ SPT reactivity ↑ lung function
Eifan et al., 2010 [51]	RCT	HDM	5–10	32/16	24	↓ asthma symptoms ↓ medication score ↓ VAS ↓ sIgE and SPT for HDM
Keles et al., 2011 [52]	RCT	HDM	5–12	48/12	18	↓ asthma attacks, ↓ inhaled steroid dosage
Yukselen et al., 2012 [53]	RDBPC	HDM	6–14	21/10	12	↓ asthma symptoms ↓ medication use ↓ VAS ↓ sIgE and SPT for HDM
Rolinck-Werninghaus et al., 2004 [55]	RDBPC	Grass	3–14	20/19	32	↓ medication score
Bufe et al., 2009 [54]	RDBPC	Grass	5–16	126/127	10	↓ asthma symptoms
Stelmach et al., 2009 [56]	RDBPC	Grass	6–17	25/25	24	↓ asthma symptoms ↑ FEV1 ↓ medication use
Vourdas et al., 1998 [58]	RDBPC	Olive	7–17	33/29	24	↓ asthma symptoms

Table 1. *Cont.*

Author, Year	Trial	Allergen Extract	Age (Years)	Population (Active/Controls)	AIT Duration (Months)	Outcome
La Rosa et al., 1999 [31]	RDBPC	Parietaria	6–14	20/21	24	↓ rhinitis symptoms ↓ SPT ↑ sIgG4
Pajno et al., 2004 [59]	RDBPC	Parietaria	8–14	15/15	24	↓ bronchial hyperreactivity
Valovirta et al., 2006 [30]	RDBPC	Tree pollen	5–15	59/29	17	↓ symptoms ↓ medication use
Nolte et al., 2020 [61]	RDBPC	Ragweed	5–17	513/512	7	↓ asthma symptoms ↓ short-acting beta2-agonist use

DBPC, double-blind placebo-controlled; EBC, exhaled breath condensate; ECP, eosinophil cationic protein; FEV1, forced expiratory volume in the 1st second; HDM, house dust mite; IL-13, interleukin 13; PEF, peak expiratory flow; PRL, prolactin; RCT, randomized controlled study; SPT, skin prick test; VAS, visual analog scale; ↑, increased; ↓, diminished.

7. Mold and Pet Allergens

The role of immunotherapy for allergens different from pollen and HDM is debated in asthma therapy. Mold allergies are frequent, especially in the Mediterranean area where 20% of allergic patients are sensitized [62,63]. Sensitization to molds is associated with a more severe progression of asthma [64]. AIT has been performed for *Alternaria* and *Cladosporium* but the use is limited by difficulty in obtaining a standardized allergen extract. Despite some evidence suggesting that specific AIT has a positive effect on respiratory symptoms, high quality studies are lacking. Several limitations characterize the available studies: many trials include both children and adults, small samples, absence of a placebo group. A meta-analysis [65] including nine randomized controlled studies (RCT) highlighted that low-strength evidence suggests that mold AIT is effective for respiratory symptoms. Just one of the selected studies was performed in children using *Alternaria* SCIT and it found an improvement of the symptom–medication score and the quality of life starting from the second year of administration. Regarding SLIT, in an RDBPCT [66], 27 patients aged 14–44 years with allergic rhinitis with or without intermittent asthma were treated with *Alternaria* SLIT. A significant reduction in symptoms, medication intake, and skin test reactivity in the active group was reported. So, the role of *Alternaria* immunotherapy in children remains unclear. There is little evidence for the use of SCIT but not of SLIT for *Cladosporium*.

To our knowledge, there is no study conducted exclusively on pediatric population regarding SLIT for animal dander [67]. An RDBPCT by Alvarez-Cuesta et al. [68] enrolling adolescents and adults with allergic rhinitis with or without asthma to cat dander showed an improvement of nasal symptoms but not of the bronchial symptom score, and a decreased PEF response to cat exposure in the SLIT group compared to the placebo group. Studies on SLIT for dander of other furry animals are lacking. Currently, high-quality studies on SCIT with dog allergen extracts have failed in asthmatic children [69].

8. The Effects of SLIT on Asthma Prevention

Allergic rhinitis predicts the development of asthma in children [70,71]. It has been documented that a three-year course of SCIT significantly reduced the occurrence of asthma in children with rhinitis caused by grass and/or birch pollen after 3 and 10 years [72]. Subsequently, two open RCT found that grass SLIT drops [73] and HDM, grass, birch SLIT drops [74] significantly reduced the risk of onset of asthma in children with allergic rhinitis after a course of 3 years. More recently, a large RDBPCT [75] has showed that grass SLIT tablets prevented respiratory symptoms and the use of asthma medication in children with allergic rhinitis. The results of the studies are reported in Table 2. In a large retrospective real-life study, Zielen [76] showed for the tablet formulation in patients >5 years of age that the relative risk reduction of asthma occurrence was around 30% during the treatment and around 40% during the follow-up. There is no evidence that AIT prevents development of new additional allergic sensitization in sensitized patients [77].

Table 2. Studies on the long-term effect and preventive role of SLIT in allergic children.

Author, Year	Type of Study	Aim of the Study	Allergen Extract	Patients' Age (y)	Population (Total Patients, Active/Control Groups)	AIT Duration (Months)	Main Results
Novembre et al., 2004 [73]	RCT	Determine whether SLIT is effective in reducing ocular and nasal symptoms and the development of asthma in allergic children	Grass pollen	5–14	113 (54/59)	4	SLIT ↓ seasonal allergic rhinitis symptoms and ↓ the development of seasonal asthma
Marogna et al., 2008 [74]	RCT	Evaluate the clinical and preventive effects of SLIT in allergic children	Grass pollen	5–17	216 (144/72)	36	SLIT reduced the onset of new sensitizations and mild persistent asthma and ↓ bronchial hyperreactivity
Valovirta et al., 2018 [75]	RDBPC	Investigate the effect of grass SLIT on the risk of developing asthma	Grass pollen	5–12	812 (398/414)	36	SLIT ↓ the risk of experiencing asthma symptoms or using asthma medication ↓Total IgE, ↓sIgE and SPT for grass pollen

RCT, randomized controlled study, SPT, skin prick test.

9. Safety

SLIT has been shown to be a safe treatment in many clinical trials and post-marketing surveys both in adults and in children, as well as in pre-school aged children [78], in children with allergic rhinitis or controlled asthma [79–83] (Table 3). SLIT has a better safety profile compared with SCIT and it can be safely given at home. Several RDBPCTs showed that the rate of systemic adverse events did not differ between the placebo and the active group [79]. Mild local adverse reactions are commonly reported [84]. They disappear within a few days of treatment. The well-known adverse events of SLIT mainly consist of oral itching or swelling, lip edema, throat pruritus, stomach ache. They are easily contained by transitorily diminishing the dose or antihistamine premedication for several weeks. Systemic reactions and asthma exacerbations are not common [79], while anaphylaxis has been reported anecdotally [85,86], and no fatality has been registered. A very low percentage of patients discontinues SLIT because of side effects [20,39,85]. Contraindications include serious immune-associated diseases (e.g., severe immunodeficiencies), malignancies, chronic and disabling diseases (e.g., major cardiovascular disease, chronic infections, severe psychological disorders) [87]. Beta-blocker treatment is a relative contraindication. If uncontrolled asthma is a risk factor for developing serious adverse events in response to SCIT [69,88], it is reasonable to infer that in these patients SLIT is contraindicated [85]. The daily SLIT dose should temporarily not be given in the following circumstances: bronchospasm, acute febrile illness, oral injury or ulceration (e.g., dentalextraction, aphtae).

Table 3. Studies evaluating safety of sublingual immunotherapy in young children.

Author, Year	Allergen Extract	Age (Year)	Population (Total Patients, Active/Control Groups If Applicable)	AIT Duration (Months)	Main Results
Agostinis et al., 2004 [81]	HDM, grass	1–3	36	12–36	SLIT can be safely administered to very young children.
Di Rienzo et al., 2005 [78]	Various	3–5	126	24	SLIT is safe in children under the age of 5 years.
Fiocchi et al., 2005 [82]	Various	3–6	65	12	High-dose immunotherapy in children younger than 5 years is as safe as in older children.

10. Indications

The impact of SLIT on asthma is often assessed as a secondary outcome in studies on IgE-mediated allergic rhinitis. So, SLIT should be used in children with controlled mild and moderate asthma [16] or controlled severe asthma [69] associated with allergic rhinoconjunctivitis. There is a conditional recommendation on the use of SLIT in children when allergic asthma is isolated because of the moderate or low quality of evidence [16] that does not allow defining a clear recommendation [89]. However, the EAACI Guidelines [2] state that the available evidence support the efficacy of HDM SLIT for pediatric asthma and recommend HDM SLIT drops for children with controlled HDM-driven allergic asthma as an add-on treatment. For other allergens, the prescription clearly depends on the product and the type of the eliciting allergen. SLIT tablets or SLIT drops with documented efficacy should be given to asthmatic children with allergy to grass, birch, or other pollens. Low-quality data support the use of SLIT in children with allergy to *Alternaria* and cat dander [69].

In polysensitized children constituting the majority of those with a pollen allergy, the molecular-based diagnosis would permit the identification of genuine sensitizers and cross-reactive panallergens [90]. The effectiveness of AIT would possibly be increased by prescribing AIT only for genuine allergens. In the pollen—food allergy syndrome [91], SLIT does not improve symptoms to cross-reacting foods. It should be carefully excluded that asthma is elicited by foods [92].

Besides the severity of manifestations, SLIT should be considered if avoidance of the identified relevant inhalant allergens is not effective or is impracticable as the most advantageous treatment set-up. SLIT should be started when pharmacotherapy is protracted, e.g., for more than 3 months, or induces side effects. The cost and the presumed adherence to SLIT are to be considered. During SLIT, children should always receive correct pharmacotherapy. SLIT efficacy should be ascertained by reduction of frequency and severity of symptoms, use of medication, and improvement of lung function. The evaluation of SLIT results should be made following at least six months of pre-coseasonal SLIT for pollen or six to twelve months for perennial allergens and SLIT can be discontinued when patients get worse. There is no absolute age limitation for SLIT administration. Even though the efficacy and safety of SLIT has been shown in children of 3 years of age, evidence is scarce [81,82,93]. Therefore, in preschool children, SLIT should be prescribed after carefully assessing risks and benefits and SLIT drops should be preferred. There are no data suggesting that children receiving SLIT are at a higher risk for the COVID-19 infection. It is recommended to carry on the administration of SLIT during the COVID-19 pandemic. Patients with suspected or confirmed infection with COVID-19 should discontinue the treatment [94]. Finally, in children with rhinoconjunctivitis caused by grass or birch, it has been shown that some SLIT products can be a feasible option not only for controlling symptoms, but also for preventing the onset of asthma [13,95]. A minimum of 3 years course is generally recommended to obtain a preventive effect [93].

11. Conclusions

SLIT is a nice example of precision medicine for allergen-driven asthma. There has been a significant progress in SLIT over the last years with introduction of new formulations. Recently approved SLIT products have been investigated in large trials, mainly in adults with asthma or in patients with allergic rhinitis, and there is a need in studies on their use in asthmatic children. Generally, SLIT appears to be safe and effective as an additional treatment in most children with controlled IgE-mediated asthma due to more common allergens. However, products differ in characteristics and efficacy. A distinction of products is necessary to avoid confusion and predict benefits.

Author Contributions: Conceptualization, C.C.; Writing—review and editing, C.C., C.M., M.P., A.S. All authors have read and agreed to the published version of the manuscript.

Funding: This review received no external funding.

Conflicts of Interest: The authors declare no conflict of interest.

References

1. Van de Griendt, E.J.; Tuut, M.K.; de Groot, H.; Brand, P.L.P. Applicability of evidence from previous systematic reviews on immunotherapy in current practice of childhood asthma treatment: A GRADE (Grading of Recommendations Assessment, Development and Evaluation) systematic review. *BMJ Open* **2017**, *7*, e016326. [CrossRef] [PubMed]
2. Agache, I.; Lau, S.; Akdis, C.A.; Smolinska, S.; Bonini, M.; Cavkaytar, O.; Flood, B.; Gajdanowicz, P.; Izuhara, K.; Kalayci, O.; et al. EAACI Guidelines on Allergen Immunotherapy: House dust mite-driven allergic asthma. *Allergy* **2019**, *74*, 855–873. [CrossRef] [PubMed]
3. Mastrorilli, C.; Posa, D.; Cipriani, F.; Caffarelli, C. Asthma and allergic rhinitis in childhood: What's new. *Pediatr. Allergy Immunol.* **2016**, *27*, 795–803. [CrossRef] [PubMed]
4. Lambrecht, B.N.; Hammad, H. The immunology of asthma. *Nat. Immunol.* **2015**, *16*, 45–56. [CrossRef]

5. Akar-Ghibril, N.; Casale, T.; Custovic, A.; Phipatanakul, W. Allergic endotypes and phenotypes of asthma. *J. Allergy Clin. Immunol. Pract.* **2020**, *8*, 429–440. [CrossRef]
6. Dhami, S.; Kakourou, A.; Asamoah, F.; Agache, I.; Lau, S.; Jutel, M.; Muraro, A.; Roberts, G.; Akdis, C.A.; Bonini, M.; et al. Allergen immunotherapy for allergic asthma: A systematic review and meta-analysis. *Allergy* **2017**, *72*, 1825–1848. [CrossRef]
7. Scadding, G.K.; Brostoff, J. Low dose sublingual therapy in patients with allergic rhinitis due to dust mite. *Clin. Allergy* **1986**, *16*, 483–491. [CrossRef]
8. Chelladurai, Y.; Suarez-Cuervo, C.; Erekosima, N.; Kim, J.M.; Ramanathan, M.; Segal, J.B.; Lin, S.Y. Effectiveness of subcutaneous versus sublingual immunotherapy for the treatment of allergic rhinoconjunctivitis and asthma: A systematic review. *J. Allergy Clin. Immunol. Pract.* **2013**, *1*, 361–369. [CrossRef]
9. Nelson, H.S.; Makatsori, M.; Calderon, M.A. Subcutaneous immunotherapy and sublingual immunotherapy: Comparative efficacy, current and potential indications, and warnings—United States versus Europe. *Immunol. Allergy Clin. N. Am.* **2016**, *36*, 13–24. [CrossRef]
10. Bousquet, J.; Lockey, R.; Malling, H.J. World Health Organization position paper: Allergen immunotherapy—Therapeutical vaccines for allergic diseases. *Allergy* **1998**, *53* (Suppl. 54), 1–15.
11. Canonica, G.W.; Cox, L.; Pawankar, R.; Baena-Cagnani, C.E.; Blaiss, M.; Bonini, S.; Bousquet, J.; Calderón, M.; Compalati, E.; Durham, S.R.; et al. Sublingual immunotherapy: World allergy organization position paper 2013 update. *World Allergy Organ. J.* **2014**, *7*, 6. [CrossRef] [PubMed]
12. Greenhawt, M.; Oppenheimer, J.; Nelson, M.; Nelson, H.; Lockey, R.; Lieberman, P.; Nowak-Wegrzyn, A.; Peters, A.; Collins, C.; Bernstein, D.I.; et al. Sublingual immunotherapy: A focused allergen immunotherapy practice parameter update. *Ann. Allergy Asthma Immunol.* **2017**, *118*, 276–282. [CrossRef] [PubMed]
13. Pajno, G.; Bernardini, R.; Peroni, D.; Arasi, S.; Martelli, A.; Landi, M.; Passalacqua, G.; Muraro, A.; La Grutta, S.; Fiocchi, A.; et al. Clinical practice recommendations for allergen-specific immunotherapy in children: The Italian consensus report. *Ital. J. Pediatr.* **2017**, *43*, 13. [CrossRef] [PubMed]
14. Roberts, G.; Pfaar, O.; Akdis, C.A.; Ansotegui, I.J.; Durham, S.R.; Gerth van Wijk, R.; Halken, S.; Larenas-Linnemann, D.; Pawankar, R.; Pitsios, C.; et al. EAACI guidelines on allergen immunotherapy: Allergic rhinoconjunctivitis. *Allergy* **2018**, *73*, 765–798. [CrossRef] [PubMed]
15. Di Rienzo, V.; Cadario, G.; Grieco, T.; Galluccio, A.G.; Caffarelli, C.; Liotta, G.; Pecora, S.; Burastero, S.E. Sublingual immunotherapy in mite-sensitized children with atopic dermatitis: A randomized, open, parallel-group study. *Ann. Allergy Asthma Immunol.* **2014**, *113*, 671–673. [CrossRef] [PubMed]
16. Jutel, M.; Agache, I.; Bonini, S.; Burks, A.W.; Calderon, M.; Canonica, W.; Cox, L.; Demoly, P.; Frew, A.J.; O'Hehir, R.; et al. International Consensus on Allergen Immunotherapy II: Mechanisms, standardization, and pharmacoeconomic. *J. Allergy Clin. Immunol.* **2016**, *137*, 358–368. [CrossRef]
17. Incorvaia, C.; Frati, F.; Sensi, L.; Riario-Sforza, G.G.; Marcucci, F. Allergic inflammation and the oral mucosa. *Recent Pat. Inflamm. Allergy Drug Discov.* **2007**, *1*, 35–38. [CrossRef]
18. Bonertz, A.; Mahler, V.; Vieths, S. Manufacturing and quality assessment of allergenic extracts for immunotherapy: State of the art. *Curr. Opin. Allergy Clin. Immunol.* **2019**, *19*, 640–645. [CrossRef]
19. Passalacqua, G.; Bagnasco, D.; Canonica, W. 30 years of sublingual immunotherapy. *Allergy* **2020**, *75*, 1107–1120. [CrossRef]
20. Cox, L.; Nelson, H.; Lockey, R.; Calabria, C.; Chacko, T.; Finegold, I.; Nelson, M.; Weber, R.; Bernstein, D.I.; Blessing-Moore, J.; et al. Allergen immunotherapy: A practice parameter third update. *J. Allergy Clin. Immunol.* **2011**, *127* (Suppl. 1), S1–S55. [CrossRef]
21. Tari, M.G.; Mancino, M.; Monti, G. Efficacy of sublingual immunotherapy in patients with rhinitis and asthma due to house dust mite. A double-blind study. *Allergol. Immunopathol.* **1990**, *18*, 277–284.
22. Hirsch, T.; Sähn, M.; Leupold, W. Double-blind placebo-controlled study of sublingual immunotherapy with house dust mite extract (D. pt.) in children. *Pediatr. Allergy Immunol.* **1997**, *8*, 21–27. [CrossRef]
23. Pajno, G.B.; Morabito, L.; Barberio, G.; Parmiani, S. Clinical and immunologic effects of long-term sublingual immunotherapy in asthmatic children sensitized to mites: A double-blind, placebo-controlled study. *Allergy* **2000**, *55*, 842–849. [CrossRef] [PubMed]
24. Bahçeciler, N.N.; Isik, U.; Barlan, I.B.; Basaran, M.M. Efficacy of sublingual immunotherapy in children with asthma and rhinitis: A double-blind, placebo-controlled study. *Pediatr. Pulmonol.* **2001**, *32*, 49–55. [CrossRef] [PubMed]

25. Ippoliti, F.; De Santis, W.; Volterrani, A.; Lenti, L.; Canitano, N.; Lucarelli, S.; Frediani, T. Immunomodulation during sublingual therapy in allergic children. *Pediatr. Allergy Immunol.* **2003**, *14*, 216–221. [CrossRef] [PubMed]
26. Lue, K.H.; Lin, Y.H.; Sun, H.L.; Lu, K.H.; Hsieh, J.C.; Chou, M.C. Clinical and immunologic effects of sublingual immunotherapy in asthmatic children sensitized to mites: A double-blind, randomized, placebo-controlled study. *Pediatr. Allergy Immunol.* **2006**, *17*, 408–415. [CrossRef]
27. Niu, C.K.; Chen, W.Y.; Huang, J.L.; Lue, K.H.; Wang, J.Y. Efficacy of sublingual immunotherapy with high-dose mite extracts in asthma: A multi-center, double-blind, randomized, and placebo-controlled study in Taiwan. *Respir. Med.* **2006**, *100*, 1374–1383. [CrossRef]
28. Pham-Thi, N.; Scheinmann, P.; Fadel, R.; Combebias, A.; Andre, C. Assessment of sublingual immunotherapy efficacy in children with house dust mite-induced allergic asthma optimally controlled by pharmacologic treatment and mite-avoidance measures. *Pediatr. Allergy Immunol.* **2007**, *18*, 47–57. [CrossRef]
29. Marcucci, F.; Sensi, L.; Di Cara, G.; Incorvaia, C.; Frati, F. Dose dependence of immunological response to sublingual immunotherapy. *Allergy* **2005**, *60*, 952–956. [CrossRef]
30. Valovirta, E.; Jacobsen, L.; Ljørring, C.; Koivikko, A.; Savolainen, J. Clinical efficacy and safety of sublingual immunotherapy with tree pollen extract in children. *Allergy* **2006**, *61*, 1177–1183. [CrossRef]
31. La Rosa, M.; Ranno, C.; André, C.; Carat, F.; Tosca, M.A.; Canonica, G.W. Double-blind placebo-controlled evaluation of sublingual-swallow immunotherapy with standardized Parietaria judaica extract in children with allergic rhinoconjunctivitis. *J. Allergy Clin. Immunol.* **1999**, *104*, 425–432. [CrossRef]
32. Lombardi, C.; Braga, M.; Incorvaia, C.; Senna, G.; Canonica, G.W.; Passalacqua, G. Administration regimens for sublingual immunotherapy. What do we know? *Allergy* **2009**, *64*, 849–854. [CrossRef]
33. Muraro, A.; Roberts, G.; Halken, S.; Agache, I.; Angier, E.; Fernandez-Rivas, M.; Gerth van Wijk, R.; Jutel, M.; Lau, S.; Pajno, G.; et al. EAACI guidelines on allergen immunotherapy: Executive statement. *Allergy* **2018**, *73*, 739–743. [CrossRef] [PubMed]
34. Penagos, M.; Durham, S.R. Duration of allergen immunotherapy for inhalant allergy. *Curr. Opin. Allergy Clin. Immunol.* **2019**, *19*, 594–605. [CrossRef] [PubMed]
35. Pfaar, O.; Alvaro, M.; Cardona, V.; Hamelmann, E.; Mösges, R.; Kleine-Tebbe, J. Clinical trials in allergen immunotherapy: Current concepts and future needs. *Allergy* **2018**, *73*, 1775–1783. [CrossRef]
36. Marogna, M.; Spadolini, I.; Massolo, A.; Canonica, G.W.; Passalacqua, G. Long-lasting effects of sublingual immunotherapy according to its duration: A 15-year prospective study. *J. Allergy Clin. Immunol.* **2010**, *126*, 969–975. [CrossRef]
37. De Groot, E.P.; Nijkamp, A.; Duiverman, E.J.; Brand, P.L. Allergic rhinitis is associated with poor asthma control, mostly if topic corticosteroid treatment is uneffective. *Thorax* **2012**, *67*, 582–587. [CrossRef]
38. Shamssain, M.H.; Shamsian, N. Prevalence and severity of asthma, rhinitis, and atopic eczema in 13- to 14-year-old school children from the northeast of England. *Ann. Allergy Asthma Immunol.* **2001**, *86*, 428–432. [CrossRef]
39. Rice, J.L.; Diette, G.B.; Suarez-Cuervo, C.; Brigham, E.P.; Lin, S.Y.; Ramanathan, M.; Robinson, K.A.; Azar, A. Allergen-specific immunotherapy in the treatment of pediatric asthma: A systematic review. *Pediatrics* **2018**, *141*, e20173833. [CrossRef]
40. Global Initiative for Asthma. Global Strategy for Asthma Management and Prevention (2020 Update). Available online: https://ginasthma.org/gina-reports/ (accessed on 21 September 2020).
41. Nieto, A.; Mazon, A.; Pamies, R.; Bruno, M.; Navarro, M.; Montanes, A. Sublingual immunotherapy for allergic respiratory diseases: An evaluation of meta-analyses. *J. Allergy Clin. Immunol.* **2009**, *124*, 157–161. [CrossRef]
42. Penagos, M.; Passalacqua, G.; Compalati, E.; Baena-Cagnani, C.E.; Orozco, S.; Pedroza, A.; Canonica, G.W. Metaanalysis of the efficacy of sublingual immunotherapy in the treatment of allergic asthma in pediatric patients, 3 to 18 years of age. *Chest* **2008**, *133*, 599–609. [CrossRef]
43. Kim, J.M.; Lin, S.Y.; Suarez-Cuervo, C.; Chelladurai, Y.; Ramanathan, M.; Segal, J.B.; Erekosima, N. Allergen-specific immunotherapy for pediatric asthma and rhinoconjunctivitis: A systematic review. *Pediatrics* **2013**, *131*, 1155–1167. [CrossRef] [PubMed]
44. Virchow, J.C.; Backer, V.; Kuna, P.; Prieto, L.; Nolte, H.; Villesen, H.H.; Ljørring, C.; Riis, B.; de Blay, F. Efficacy of a house dust mite sublingual allergen immunotherapy tablet in adults with allergic asthma: A randomized clinical trial. *JAMA* **2016**, *315*, 1715–1725. [CrossRef]

45. Nolte, H.; Maloney, J.; Nelson, H.S.; Bernstein, D.I.; Lu, S.; Li, Z.; Kaur, A.; Zieglmayer, P.; Zieglmayer, R.; Lemell, P.; et al. Onset and dose-related efficacy of house dust mite sublingual immunotherapy tablets in an environmental exposure chamber. *J. Allergy Clin. Immunol.* **2015**, *135*, 1494–1501. [CrossRef] [PubMed]
46. Mosbech, H.; Deckelmann, R.; de Blay, F.; Pastorello, E.A.; Trebas-Pietras, E.; Andres, L.P.; Malcus, I.; Ljørring, C.; Canonica, G.W. Standardized quality (SQ) house dust mite sublingual immunotherapy tablet (ALK) reduces inhaled corticosteroid use while maintaining asthma control: A randomized, double-blind, placebo controlled trial. *J. Allergy Clin. Immunol.* **2014**, *134*, 568–575. [CrossRef] [PubMed]
47. Bousquet, J.; Scheinmann, P.; Guinnepain, M.T.; Perrin-Fayolle, M.; Sauvaget, J.; Tonnel, A.B.; Pauli, G.; Caillaud, D.; Dubost, R.; Leynadier, F.; et al. Sublingual-swallow immunotherapy (SLIT) in patients with asthma due to house-dust mites: A double-blind, placebo-controlled study. *Allergy* **1999**, *54*, 249–260. [CrossRef] [PubMed]
48. Wang, L.; Yin, J.; Fadel, R.; Montagut, A.; de Beaumont, O.; Devillier, P. House dust mite sublingual immunotherapy is safe and appears to be effective in moderate, persistent asthma. *Allergy* **2014**, *69*, 1181–1188. [CrossRef]
49. Mosbech, H.; Canonica, G.W.; Backer, V.; de Blay, F.; Klimek, L.; Broge, L.; Ljørring, C. SQ house dust mite sublingually administered immunotherapy tablet (ALK) improves allergic rhinitis in patients with house dust mite allergic asthma and rhinitis symptoms. *Ann. Allergy Asthma Immunol.* **2015**, *114*, 134–140. [CrossRef]
50. De Blay, F.; Kuna, P.; Prieto, L.; Ginko, T.; Seitzberg, D.; Riis, B.; Canonica, G.W. SQ HDM SLIT-tablet (ALK) in treatment of asthma–post hoc results from a randomised trial. *Respir. Med.* **2014**, *108*, 1430–1437. [CrossRef]
51. Eifan, A.O.; Akkoc, T.; Yildiz, A.; Keles, S.; Ozdemir, C.; Bahceciler, N.N.; Barlan, I.B. Clinical efficacy and immunological mechanisms of sublingual and subcutaneous immunotherapy in asthmatic/rhinitis children sensitized to house dust mite: An open randomized controlled trial. *Clin. Exp. Allergy* **2010**, *40*, 922–932. [CrossRef]
52. Keles, S.; Karakoc-Aydiner, E.; Ozen, A.; Izgi, A.G.; Tevetoglu, A.; Akkoc, T.; Bahceciler, N.N.; Barlan, I. A novel approach in allergen-specific immunotherapy: Combination of sublingual and subcutaneous routes. *J. Allergy Clin. Immunol.* **2011**, *128*, 808–815. [CrossRef] [PubMed]
53. Yukselen, A.; Kendirli, S.G.; Yilmaz, M.; Altintas, D.U.; Karacoc, G.B. Effect of one-year subcutaneous and sublingual immunotherapy on clinical and laboratory parameters in children with rhinitis and asthma: A randomized, placebo-controlled, double-blind, double-dummy study. *Int. Arch. Allergy Immunol.* **2012**, *157*, 288–298. [CrossRef] [PubMed]
54. Bufe, A.; Eberle, P.; Franke-Beckmann, E.; Funck, J.; Kimmig, M.; Klimek, L.; Knecht, R.; Stephan, V.; Tholstrup, B.; Weisshaar, C.; et al. Safety and efficacy in children of an SQ-standardized grass allergen tablet for sublingual immunotherapy. *J. Allergy Clin. Immunol.* **2009**, *123*, 167–173. [CrossRef] [PubMed]
55. Rolinck-Werninghaus, C.; Wolf, H.; Liebke, C.; Baars, J.C.; Lange, J.; Kopp, M.V.; Hammermann, J.; Leupold, W.; Bartels, P.; Gruebl, A.; et al. A prospective, randomized, double-blind, placebo-controlled multi-centre study on the efficacy and safety of sublingual immunotherapy (SLIT) in children with seasonal allergic rhinoconjunctivitis to grass pollen. *Allergy* **2004**, *59*, 1285–1293. [CrossRef] [PubMed]
56. Stelmach, I.; Kaczmarek-Woźniak, J.; Majak, P.; Oszłowiek-Chlebna, M.; Jerzynska, A. Efficacy and safety of high-doses sublingual immunotherapy in ultra-rush scheme in children allergic to grass pollen. *Clin. Exp. Allergy* **2009**, *39*, 401–408. [CrossRef] [PubMed]
57. Devillier, P.; Molimard, M.; Ansolabehere, X.; Bardoulat, I.; Coulombel, N.; Maurel, F.; Le Jeunne, P.; Demoly, P. Immunotherapy with grass pollen tablets reduces medication dispensing for allergic rhinitis and asthma: A retrospective database study in France. *Allergy* **2019**, *74*, 1317–1326. [CrossRef] [PubMed]
58. Vourdas, D.; Syrigou, E.; Potamianou, P.; Carat, F.; Batard, T.; André, C.; Papageorgiou, P.S. Double-blind placebo-controlled evaluation of sublingual-swallow immunotherapy with standardized olive pollen extract in pediatric patients with allergic rhinoconjunctivitis and mild asthma due a olive pollen sensitization. *Allergy* **1998**, *53*, 662–672. [CrossRef]
59. Pajno, G.; Passalacqua, G.; Vita, D.; Permiani, S.; Barberio, G. Sublingual immunotherapy abrogates seasonal bronchial hyperresponsiveness in children with Parietaria-induced respiratory allergy: A randomized controlled trial. *Allergy* **2004**, *59*, 883–887. [CrossRef]

60. Biedermann, T.; Kuna, P.; Panzner, P.; Valovirta, E.; Andersson, M.; de Blay, F.; Thrane, D.; Jacobsen, S.H.; Stage, B.S.; Winther, L. The SQ tree SLIT-tablet is highly effective and well tolerated: Results from a randomized, double-blind, placebo-controlled phase III trial. *J. Allergy Clin. Immunol.* **2019**, *143*, 1058–1066. [CrossRef]
61. Nolte, H.; Bernstein, D.I.; Nelson, H.S.; Ellis, A.K.; Kleine-Tebbe, J.; Lu, S. Efficacy and safety of ragweed slit-tablet in children with allergic rhinoconjunctivitis in a randomized, placebo-controlled trial. *J. Allergy Clin. Immunol Pract.* **2020**, *8*, 2322–2331.e5. [CrossRef]
62. Bousquet, P.J.; Chinn, S.; Janson, C.; Kogevinas, M.; Burney, P.; Jarvis, D. Geographical variation in the prevalence of positive skin tests to environmental aeroallergens in the European Community Respiratory Health Survey, I. *Allergy* **2007**, *62*, 301–309. [CrossRef]
63. D'Amato, G.; Chatzigeorgiou, G.; Corsico, R.; Gioulekas, D.; Jäger, L.; Jäger, S.; Kontou-Fili, K.; Kouridakis, S.; Liccardi, G.; Meriggi, A.; et al. Evaluation of the prevalence of skin prick test positivity to Alternaria and Cladosporium in patients with suspected respiratory allergy. A European multicenter study promoted by the Subcommittee on Aerobiology and Environmental Aspects of Inhalant Allergens of the European Academy of Allergology and Clinical Immunology. *Allergy* **1997**, *52*, 711–716. [PubMed]
64. Larenas-Linnemann, D.; Baxi, S.; Phipatanakul, W.; Portnoy, J.M. Environmental Allergens Workgroup. Clinical evaluation and management of patients with suspected fungus sensitivity. *J. Allergy Clin. Immunol. Pract.* **2016**, *4*, 405–414. [CrossRef]
65. Di Bona, D.; Frisenda, F.; Albanesi, M.; Di Lorenzo, G.; Caiaffa, M.F.; Macchia, L. Efficacy and safety of allergen immunotherapy in patients with allergy to molds: A systematic review. *Clin. Exp. Allergy* **2018**, *48*, 1391–1401. [CrossRef] [PubMed]
66. Cortellini, G.; Spadolini, I.; Patella, V.; Fabbri, E.; Santucci, A.; Severino, M.; Corvetta, A.; Canonica, G.W.; Passalacqua, G. Sublingual immunotherapy for Alternaria induced allergic rhinitis: A randomized placebo-controlled trial. *Ann. Allergy Asthma Immunol.* **2010**, *105*, 382–386. [CrossRef] [PubMed]
67. Pfaar, O.; Bachert, C.; Bufe, A.; Buhl, R.; Ebner, C.; Eng, P.; Friedrichs, F.; Fuchs, T.; Hamelmann, E.; Hartwig-Bade, D.; et al. Guideline on allergen-specific immunotherapy in IgE-mediated allergic diseases: S2k Guideline of the German Society for Allergology and Clinical Immunology (DGAKI), the Society for Pediatric Allergy and Environmental Medicine (GPA), the Medical Association of German Allergologists (AeDA), the Austrian Society for Allergy and Immunology (ÖGAI), the Swiss Society for Allergy and Immunology (SGAI), the German Society of Dermatology (DDG), the German Society of Oto- Rhino-Laryngology, Head and Neck Surgery (DGHNO-KHC), the German Society of Pediatrics and Adolescent Medicine (DGKJ), the Society for Pediatric Pneumology (GPP), the German Respiratory Society (DGP), the German Association of ENT Surgeons (BV-HNO), the Professional Federation of Paediatricians and Youth Doctors (BVKJ), the Federal Association of Pulmonologists (BDP) and the German Dermatologists Association (BVDD). *Allergo J. Int.* **2014**, *23*, 282–319. [PubMed]
68. Alvarez-Cuesta, E.; Berges Gimeno, P.; Mancebo, E.G.; Fernandez-Caldas, E.; Cuesta-Herranz, J.; Casanovas, M. Sublingual immunotherapy with a standardized cat dander extract: Evaluation of efficacy in a double blind placebo controlled study. *Allergy* **2007**, *62*, 810–817. [CrossRef]
69. Alvaro-Lozano, M.; Akdis, C.A.; Akdis, M.; Alviani, C.; Angier, E.; Arasi, S.; Arzt-Gradwohl, L.; Barber, D.; Bazire, R.; Cavkaytor, O.; et al. Allergen Immunotherapy in Children User's Guide. *Pediatr. Allergy Immunol.* **2020**, *31* (Suppl. 25), 1–101. [CrossRef]
70. Roberts, G.; Xatzipsalti, M.; Borrego, L.M.; Custovic, A.; Halken, S.; Hellings, P.W.; Papadopoulos, N.G.; Rotiroti, G.; Scadding, G.; Timmermans, F.; et al. Paediatric rhinitis: Position paper of the European Academy of Allergy and Clinical Immunology. *Allergy* **2013**, *68*, 1102–1116. [CrossRef]
71. Burgess, J.A.; Walters, E.H.; Byrnes, G.B.; Matheson, M.C.; Jenkins, M.A.; Wharton, C.L.; Johns, D.P.; Abramson, M.J.; Hopper, J.L.; Dharmage, S.C. Childhood allergic rhinitis predicts asthma incidence and persistence to middle age: A longitudinal study. *J. Allergy Clin. Immunol.* **2007**, *120*, 863–869. [CrossRef]
72. Jacobsen, L.; Niggemann, B.; Dreborg, S.; Ferdousi, H.A.; Halken, S.; Høst, A.; Koivikko, A.; Norberg, L.A.; Valovirta, E.; Wahn, U.; et al. Specific immunotherapy has long-term preventive effect of seasonal and perennial asthma: 10-year followup on the PAT study. *Allergy* **2007**, *62*, 943–948. [CrossRef] [PubMed]
73. Novembre, E.; Galli, E.; Landi, F.; Caffarelli, C.; Pifferi, M.; De marco, E.; Burastero, S.E.; Calori, G.; Benetti, L.; Bonazza, P.; et al. Coseasonal sublingual immunotherapy reduces the development of asthma in children with allergic rhinoconjunctivitis. *J. Allergy Clin. Immunol.* **2004**, *114*, 851–857. [CrossRef] [PubMed]

74. Marogna, M.; Tomassetti, D.; Bernasconi, A.; Colombo, F.; Massolo, A.; Di Rienzo Businco, A.; Canonica, G.W.; Passalacqua, G.; Tripodi, S. Preventive effects of sublingual immunotherapy in childhood: An open randomized controlled study. *Ann. Allergy Asthma Immunol.* **2008**, *101*, 206–211. [CrossRef]
75. Valovirta, E.; Petersen, T.H.; Piotrowska, T.; Laursen, M.K.; Andersen, J.S.; Sørensen, H.F.; Klink, R.; GAP Investigators. Results from the 5-year SQ grass sublingual immunotherapy tablet asthma prevention (GAP) trial in children with grass pollen allergy. *J. Allergy Clin. Immunol.* **2018**, *141*, 529–538. [CrossRef] [PubMed]
76. Zielen, S.; Devillier, P.; Heinrich, J.; Richter, H.; Wahn, U. Sublingual immunotherapy provides long-term relief in allergic rhinitis and reduces the risk of asthma: A retrospective, real-word database analysis. *Allergy* **2018**, *73*, 165–177. [CrossRef]
77. Kristiansen, M.; Dhami, S.; Netuveli, G.; Halken, S.; Muraro, A.; Roberts, G.; Larenas-Linnemann, D.; Calderon, M.A.; Penagos, M.; Du Toit, G.; et al. Allergen immunotherapy for the prevention of allergy: A systematic review and meta-analysis. *Pediatr. Allergy Immunol.* **2017**, *28*, 18–29. [CrossRef]
78. Rienzo, V.D.; Minelli, M.; Musarra, A.; Sambugaro, R.; Pecora, S.; Canonica, W.G.; Passalacqua, G. Post-marketing survey on the safety of sublingual immunotherapy in children below the age of 5 years. *Clin. Exp. Allergy* **2005**, *35*, 560–564. [CrossRef]
79. Rodrıguez Del Rıo, P.; Vidal, C.; Just, J.; Tabar, A.I.; Sanchez-Machin, I.; Eberle, P.; Borja, J.; Bubel, P.; Pfaar, O.; Demoly, P.; et al. The European Survey on Adverse Systemic Reactions in Allergen Immunotherapy (EASSI): A paediatric assessment. *Pediatr. Allergy Immunol.* **2017**, *28*, 60–70. [CrossRef]
80. Passalacqua, G.; Nowak-Wegrzyn, A.; Canonica, G.W. Local side effects of sublingual and oral immunotherapy. *J. Allergy Clin. Immunol. Pract.* **2017**, *5*, 13–21. [CrossRef]
81. Agostinis, F.; Tellarini, L.; Canonica, G.W.; Falagiani, P.; Passalacqua, G. Safety of sublingual immunotherapy with a monomeric allergoid in very young children. *Allergy* **2005**, *60*, 133. [CrossRef]
82. Fiocchi, A.; Pajno, G.; La Grutta, S.; Pezzuto, F.; Incorvaia, C.; Sensi, L.; Marcucci, F.; Frati, F. Safety of sublingual-swallow immunotherapy in children aged 3 to 7 years. *Ann. Allergy Asthma Immunol.* **2005**, *95*, 254–258. [CrossRef]
83. Passalacqua, G.; Guerra, L.; Pasquali, M.; Lombardi, C.; Canonica, G.W. Efficacy and safety of sublingual immunotherapy. *Ann. Allergy Asthma Immunol.* **2004**, *93*, 3–12. [CrossRef]
84. Kleine-Tebbe, J.; Ribel, M.; Herold, D.A. Safety of a SQ-standardised grass allergen tablet for sublingual immunotherapy: A randomized, placebo-controlled trial. *Allergy* **2006**, *61*, 181–184. [CrossRef]
85. Calderon, M.A.; Simons, F.E.R.; Malling, H.J.; Lockey, R.F.; Moingeon, P.; Demoly, P. Sublingual allergen immunotherapy: Mode of action and its relationship with the safety profile. *Allergy* **2012**, *67*, 302–311. [CrossRef] [PubMed]
86. Duric-Filipovic, I.; Caminati, M.; Kostic, G.; Filipovic, D.; Zivkovic, Z. Allergen specific sublingual immunotherapy in children with asthma and allergic rhinitis. *World J. Pediatr.* **2016**, *12*, 283–290. [CrossRef]
87. Pitsios, C.; Demoly, P.; Bilo, M.B.; Gerth van Wijk, R.; Pfaar, O.; Sturm, G.J.; Rodriguez del Rio, P.; Tsoumani, M.; Gawlik, R.; Paraskevopoulos, G.; et al. Clinical contraindications to allergen immunotherapy: An EAACI position paper. *Allergy* **2015**, *70*, 897–909. [CrossRef]
88. Reid, M.J.; Lockey, R.F.; Turkeltaub, P.C.; Platts-Mills, T.A. Survey of fatalities from skin testing and immunotherapy 1985–1989. *J. Allergy Clin. Immunol.* **1993**, *92*, 6–15. [CrossRef]
89. Normansell, R.; Kew, K.M.; Bridgman, A.L. Sublingual immunotherapy for asthma. *Cochrane Database Syst. Rev.* **2015**, *8*, CD011293. [CrossRef]
90. Cipriani, F.; Mastrorilli, C.; Tripodi, S.; Ricci, G.; Perna, S.; Panetta, V.; Asero, R.; Dondi, A.; Bianchi, A.; Maiello, N.; et al. Diagnostic relevance of IgE sensitization profiles to eight recombinant Phleum pratense molecules. *Allergy* **2018**, *73*, 673–682. [CrossRef] [PubMed]
91. Mastrorilli, C.; Cardinale, F.; Giannetti, A.; Caffarelli, C. Pollen-food allergy syndrome: A not so rare disease in childhood. *Medicina (Kaunas)* **2019**, *55*, 641. [CrossRef] [PubMed]
92. Caffarelli, C.; Garrubba, M.; Greco, C.; Mastrorilli, C.; Povesi Dascola, C. Asthma and food allergy in children: Is there a connection or interaction? *Front. Pediatr.* **2016**, *4*, 34. [CrossRef] [PubMed]
93. Cantani, A.; Arcese, G.; Lucenti, P.; Gagliesi, D.; Bartolucci, M. A three-year prospective study of specific immunotherapy to inhalant allergens: Evidence of safety and efficacy in 300 children with allergic asthma. *J. Investig. Allergol. Clin. Immunol.* **1997**, *7*, 90–97. [PubMed]

94. Cardinale, F.; Ciprandi, G.; Barberi, R.; Bernardini, R.; Caffarelli, C.; Calvani, M.; Cavagni, C.; Galli, E.; Minasi, D.; del Giudice, M.M.; et al. Consensus statement of the Italian society of pediatric allergy and immunology for the pragmatic management of children and adolescents with allergic or immunological diseases during the COVID-19 pandemic. *Ital. J. Pediatr.* **2020**, *46*, 84. [CrossRef]
95. Halken, S.; Larenas-Linnemann, D.; Roberts, G.; Moises, A.; Calderón, M.A.; Angier, E.; Pfaar, O.; Ryan, D.; Agache, I.; Ansotegui, I.J.; et al. EAACI guidelines on allergen immunotherapy: Prevention of allergy. *Pediatr. Allergy Immunol.* **2017**, *28*, 728–745. [CrossRef] [PubMed]

Publisher's Note: MDPI stays neutral with regard to jurisdictional claims in published maps and institutional affiliations.

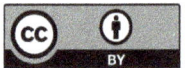

© 2020 by the authors. Licensee MDPI, Basel, Switzerland. This article is an open access article distributed under the terms and conditions of the Creative Commons Attribution (CC BY) license (http://creativecommons.org/licenses/by/4.0/).

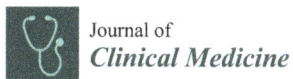

Review

Which Child with Asthma is a Candidate for Biological Therapies?

Andrew Bush

Imperial College & Royal Brompton Harefield NHS Foundation Trust, London SW£ dNP, UK; a.bush@imperial.ac.uk; Tel.: +44-207-351-8232

Received: 17 March 2020; Accepted: 22 April 2020; Published: 24 April 2020

Abstract: In asthmatic adults, monoclonals directed against Type 2 airway inflammation have led to major improvements in quality of life, reductions in asthma attacks and less need for oral corticosteroids. The paediatric evidence base has lagged behind. All monoclonals currently available for children are anti-eosinophilic, directed against the T helper (TH2) pathway. However, in children and in low and middle income settings, eosinophils may have important beneficial immunological actions. Furthermore, there is evidence that paediatric severe asthma may not be TH2 driven, phenotypes may be less stable than in adults, and adult biomarkers may be less useful. Children being evaluated for biologicals should undergo a protocolised assessment, because most paediatric asthma can be controlled with low dose inhaled corticosteroid if taken properly and regularly. For those with severe therapy resistant asthma, and refractory asthma which cannot be addressed, the two options if they have TH2 inflammation are omalizumab and mepolizumab. There is good evidence of efficacy for omalizumab, particularly in those with multiple asthma attacks, but only paediatric safety, not efficacy, data for mepolizumab. There is an urgent need for efficacy data in children, as well as data on biomarkers to guide therapy, if the right children are to be treated with these powerful new therapies.

Keywords: airway eosinophilia; blood eosinophil count; omalizumab; mepolizumab; exhaled nitric oxide; induced sputum; allergic sensitization

1. Introduction

The purpose of this review is to give a clinically focused update on the approach to the child with asthma for whom the prescription of a biologic is being considered (omalizumab or mepolizumab, the only ones currently licensed in children), in order to appropriately select those children who need these expensive and invasive medications, to highlight the important differences between adult and paediatric severe asthma with regard to the use of biologicals and to summarise the paediatric biologic data currently published.

The *Lancet* asthma commission has highlighted that the word "asthma" is an umbrella term comprising numerous endotypes [1]. Personalised asthma medicine was first practiced by the late Dr Harry Morrow-Brown, who used his medical school microscope to show that only those patients with sputum eosinophilia responded to prednisolone and inhaled beclomethasone. This meant that two of the most effective asthma therapies that we have were not lost. This valuable lesson, a really early attempt at personalised medicine, was lost to the asthma community in the excitement at the efficacy of inhaled corticosteroids (ICS), which were widely and often indiscriminately prescribed. When the anti-interleukin(IL)-5 monoclonal mepolizumab became available, it was again prescribed indiscriminately in adult asthma and was initially thought to be ineffective [2,3]. Fortunately, the obvious fact that anti-T-helper 2 (TH2) strategies would likely not work in non-eosinophilic asthma was appreciated, and the benefits of mepolizumab in attack prone, eosinophilic adult asthmatics was appreciated [4,5].

So as an example, the absolutely critical importance of personalised therapy has not been lost on the cystic fibrosis (CF) community. The knowledge of the different classes of CF genes [6] led to the discovery of Ivacaftor, which was dramatically effective (improved weight, lung function and quality of life, sweat chloride concentration halved) in Class III gating mutations [7]. Had Ivacaftor been given to all patients with a wet productive cough, or even all patients with CF, it would have been discarded as inactive. There is an obvious lesson here for the asthma community—unless and until we really understand pathways to disease, we are at risk of discarding important therapies.

The data and indications for mepolizumab and other biologicals has been summarised recently by the ERS/ATS Task Force, but these are largely in adults [8], for whom there have been major benefits in terms of better quality of life, fewer asthma attacks, and less requirement for oral corticosteroids. Whether the patient is eligible for an anti-Type 2 inflammation biologic is usually determined by the peripheral blood eosinophil count, which in adult studies at least, has been shown to be a good surrogate for airway eosinophilic inflammation [9]. However, even in adult studies, the correlation between a TH2 high signature in bronchial epithelial cells and elevation in blood eosinophils and exhaled nitric oxide (F_ENO) is not good [10] and periostin, now being discarded even in adult medicine, cannot be used in children because it is secreted by growing bone. So in summary, anti-TH2 strategies are deployed in adult medicine if there is an elevated blood eosinophil count, on the assumption that airway phenotypes are stable. The tacit assumption is that eosinophilia equates to TH2 pathway activation; but even in adults, non-TH2 eosinophilic phenotypes are well described in U-BIOPRED, related to genes encoding metabolic pathways, ubiquitination and mitochondrial function [11]. We discuss these and other assumptions in more detail below.

Currently, only two biologicals (omalizumab, mepolizumab) are licensed in children age six years and over for severe asthma. There are extensive paediatric omalizumab data, but for mepolizumab, extrapolation from adult studies comprise the bulk of our information; and extrapolation from adults to children is dangerous. In this review, we explore the following issues, which are highly relevant to the role of biologicals in children:

1. Is the eosinophil always the "bad guy" or could there be a down side to the aggressive, anti-eosinophil strategies which have been effective in adults?
2. Is paediatric severe, therapy resistant asthma (STRA) the same as adult disease?
3. What is a truly severe disease in childhood, in other words, is it only children with STRA who should receive these medications?
4. How should we evaluate children referred for biological therapies?
5. What are the paediatric data on the biologicals, and how do we match the right biological to the right child?

The definition of STRA combines the pharmacological criteria in Table 1 together with a failure to identify any reversible factors or co-morbidities on detailed assessment (below), in other words, uncontrolled asthma even despite all basic management being optimised. We conclude with suggestions as to how the present unsatisfactory, often non-evidence-based situation can be rectified.

2. The Eosinophil: A Janus Cell, Facing Both Ways?

The eosinophil has long been considered the effector cell in Type 2 inflammation driven asthma, but potential important beneficial roles are often not considered, and there may be developmentally important roles. Immunological effects include B-cell priming and maintenance of memory plasma cells [12,13], and antigen-presenting functions in the intestine [14]. Adipose tissue eosinophils participate in beige fat thermogenesis and glucose homeostasis through regulation of alternatively activated macrophages [15,16]. At least in murine models, there is evidence that eosinophils possess significant antiviral effects, and enhancing the eosinophilic response inhibits experimental influenza and respiratory syncytial viral infection [17].

The eosinophil is important in immunity to parasites, and this may be particularly important in low and middle income (LMIC) settings. In this context, it should be noted that the predictive power of blood eosinophil counts for monoclonal responses may be less good than in a high income setting, although this has yet to be tested due to poor availability of these medications in LMICs.

In summary, the potential beneficial roles of the eosinophil should be considered in the developmental and geographical context of the individual patient when assessing the risks and benefits of anti-IL5 therapy.

3. Adult and Paediatric STRA: Similarities and Differences

The question arises as to whether Type 2 inflammation is important in paediatric STRA. Our large series of carefully characterised children with STRA who underwent bronchoscopy showed that most, but by no means all, had airway mucosal and bronchoalveolar lavage (BAL) eosinophilia [18]. To our surprise, evidence of TH2 activation was scant. Induced sputum supernatant was positive for IL5 in only 8/41 patients; BAL was interrogated using both Luminex and Cytokine Bead Array platforms, and in the fifty samples available, ten were positive for IL4, and eight for IL5 and IL13. Immunohistochemistry demonstrated more IL5 positive mucosal cells in controls, and equal numbers of IL13 positive cells in the two groups. It was difficult to conclude that TH2 inflammation was of major importance in this group; possibly at an early stage of the disease TH2 inflammation had played a role, but the pathway is steroid sensitive and all these patients were being prescribed high-dose ICS. Our subsequent studies have focussed on the possible role of the epithelial alarmin IL33 as a steroid-resistant cytokine implicated in the pathology of STRA [19,20]. These findings are in accord with the other studies [21,22].

The USA Severe Asthma Research Program studied (BAL) supernatant and alveolar macrophages in 53 asthmatic children, of whom 31 were thought to have STRA, and 30 non-smoking adults [21]. They analysed a total of 23 cytokines and found no differences between the groups for any individual cytokine, but by using linear discriminant analysis, five cytokines were able to differentiate between mild asthma, severe asthma and healthy controls: these were growth-related oncogene (GRO), RANTES (CCL5, regulated upon activation, normal T cell expressed and presumably secreted), IL12, Interferon (IFN)-γ and IL10. They also concluded that there was no TH2 signal (nor indeed classical signature TH1 cytokines) in severe paediatric asthma.

These observations have recently been taken further in a recent manuscript from the USA [22]. This group analysed bronchoalveolar lavage (BAL) (n = 68) samples from 52 children age 0.5–17 years with STRA, not all of whom were allergic. They found that memory CCR51 TH1 cells were enriched in BAL, and many viruses and bacteria were detected. Furthermore, TH17-associated mediators (IL23, MIP 3a/CCL20) were highly expressed but TH2 cells were not prominent. TH2 cytokines were detected, and correlated with total IgE and IL5 correlated with BAL eosinophil count. IL5, IL33 and IL28A/IFNl2 were increased only in multi-sensitized children. Overall, there was a dominant TH1, not TH2 signature, with multiple bacteria and viruses being present, irrespective of allergic status.

Overall, there is considerable evidence suggesting that STRA that has been treated with high-dose ICS may, in many cases, not be a TH2-driven disease. Of course, the most important question is not whether anti-IL5 strategies should work but whether they do work. However, these data underscore the need for trials in children, and that it is not acceptable to extrapolate from adult studies.

4. Are Sputum Phenotypes Stable in Paediatric Asthma?

The supposition has been that sputum phenotypes are consistent over time in adults. In the only paper in children studying sputum phenotypes longitudinally [23], sputum phenotype changes unrelated to change in prescribed treatment were very common; 20/42 (48%) children with severe asthma exhibited more than one sputum phenotype (eosinophilic, neutrophilic, mixed, pauci-inflammatory) over a one-year period; for mild–moderate asthma, 4/17 (24%) had different phenotypes on paired sputum samples. On consideration, perhaps this is unsurprising; a sputum phenotype does not exist in isolation, but in an environment. So, for example, a child with TH2-driven asthma may be pauci-inflammatory if taking ICS regularly, become eosinophilic if adherence tails off or the child is exposed to a large allergen load (as has been seen with thunderstorm asthma [24]) and neutrophilic if the child develops a viral lower respiratory tract infection. This underscores the need to go from phenotypes to endotypes, understanding the underlying pathophysiology and directing treatment accordingly.

Are adult biomarkers relevant to children? There have been far fewer biomarker studies in children compared with adults. A Cochrane review suggested that titrating treatment to levels of $F_E NO$ reduces the burden of asthma attacks [25], and a raised $F_E NO$ is predictive of a response to omalizumab in adults [26]. Peripheral blood eosinophil count is used in adult studies as a marker of airway eosinophilia when considering anti-TH2 monoclonal antibody therapy. The INFANT study in pre-school children [27], albeit in post-hoc analyses, showed that peripheral blood eosinophil count combined with evidence of aeroallergen sensitisation, predicted response to ICS. However, in our hands, there is a poor correlation between blood and sputum eosinophil count; 76/88 (86%) of our STRA patients had a normal blood eosinophil count, of whom 64 (84%) had airway eosinophilia [28]. The most recent U-BIOPRED data have demonstrated that biomarkers for transcriptomically measured airway Type 2 inflammation are insufficiently sensitive and specific even in adults [10].

Omalizumab response in adults is also predicted by a raised blood eosinophil count [26]. In our hands, a fall in $F_E NO$ in response to intramuscular triamcinolone was the best predictor of omalizumab response, in a small study which has yet to be replicated [29].

It should also be noted that $F_E NO$ and sputum eosinophil count are not interchangeable [30]. In one longitudinal study, 79 children (51 severe, 28 mild-moderate asthma) contributed 197 paired sputum and $F_E NO$ measurements. Upper limits of normal were defined as $F_E NO \geq 20$ppb and sputum eosinophils ≥ 2.5. In the cross-sectional study, 75% pairs were concordant; longitudinally, only 53% were consistently concordant, and 7% were consistently discordant. The relationship varied over time, with some children sometimes having a high $F_E NO$ and normal sputum eosinophils, and then the reverse pattern on a subsequent visit. Adult studies have suggested that a raised sputum eosinophil count reflects IL5 activity, and a raised $F_E NO$ that of IL13 [31], but this has not been tested as a selection criterion between different monoclonal strategies, or validated in children.

In summary, it is wrong to extrapolate endotypes from adults to children; and it is wrong to assume that biomarkers which may be valuable in adults have the same value in children. There is an imperative for us to do paediatric studies.

5. What Is True STRA in Children?

It cannot be over-emphasised that most children who are referred with "severe asthma" to tertiary centres just need to get the basics right [32]. The basic management must be assessed before considering whether the child has true STRA. If a child is not responding to low-dose ICS, the correct action is not to increase the doses but to ask "Why is this child not responding to what should work?" The answer is usually not because of unusual airway pathology, but due to failure to get the basics right. This is confirmed by thee key studies, and our own data. In the BADGER study [33], very few children got additional benefit from increasing their ICS dose above fluticasone 100 mcg/day; the greatest benefit was from adding inhaled long-acting β-2 agonists (salmeterol), and a few benefited from the addition of a leukotriene receptor antagonist (LTRA). A study determining whether azithromycin or montelukast was a better add-on treatment for children with uncontrolled asthma despite ICS and long-acting beta agonists ended in futility because most such patients were either not taking treatment or did not have asthma [34]. An inner city study to determine whether using $F_E NO$ to monitor asthma added value to standard guidelines was also futile because during the run-in period, when protocolised treatment was emphasised, the children improved so much that there was no real scope for further improvement [35]. Finally, we showed that at least half of all children referred to our severe asthma service just needed to get the basics right. So biological therapies are only exceptionally needed in children with asthma [32].

It is also clear that we need new concepts of severe asthma. Almost without exception, guidelines and consensus documents define severity by (usually arbitrary) levels of prescribed medication [36]. Table 1 shows the criteria used by the first ERS/ATS Task Force. The problem is that the level of prescribed medication relates only weakly to the domain of risk. Patients prescribed very low-dose medications may be at risk of a serious asthma attack, and even death, especially if they do not use the medications efficiently. This was clearly demonstrated by the UK National Review of Asthma Deaths [37], which showed that around half of asthma deaths were in those who would not have been classified as having severe asthma. The deaths were not related to difficult airway pathology, but to social and environmental factors, such as under-use of ICS [38], over-use of short-acting β-2 agonists [39], failure to attend routine asthma reviews, and frequent emergency care visits. The lesson from these data is that any definition of severe asthma based merely on levels of prescribed medication is not adequate. We also reported that most children referred for consideration of "beyond guidelines" therapy in fact only need to get the basics right [32]. Although many respond to guidance, some do not and remain at high risk. The important conclusion is that a definition of severe asthma solely based on levels of prescribed medication is inappropriate and environmental, and in particular social factors, must enter the definition even in adults; and this has particular relevance to deciding who should get biologicals (below).

Table 1. ERS/ATS Task Force definition of severe asthma [36]. The level of medication is combined with at least.

Level of Medication	Asthma Functional Deficit
Asthma which is only controlled or uncontrolled on therapy with ≥ 800 mcg/day BDP equivalent plus additional controllers (LABA, LTRA. Theophylline) or failed trials of these agents	Poor symptom control, e.g., Asthma Control Test (ACT) <20 ≥2 bursts of systemic corticosteroids (≥3 days each) in the previous year Serious exacerbations (≥1 hospitalisation or PICU stay) in the previous year Airflow limitation: FEV_1 < 80% predicted following SABA and LABA withhold

Abbreviations: ACT, asthma control test; BDP, beclomethasone diproprionate; LABA, long acting beta2 agonist; LTRA, leukotriene receptor antagonist; PICU, paediatric intensive care unit; SABA, short acting beta2 agonist.

6. How Should We Evaluate Children for Biological Therapies?

The protocols we use have been discussed in detail elsewhere [40–42], and are summarised in Figure 1.

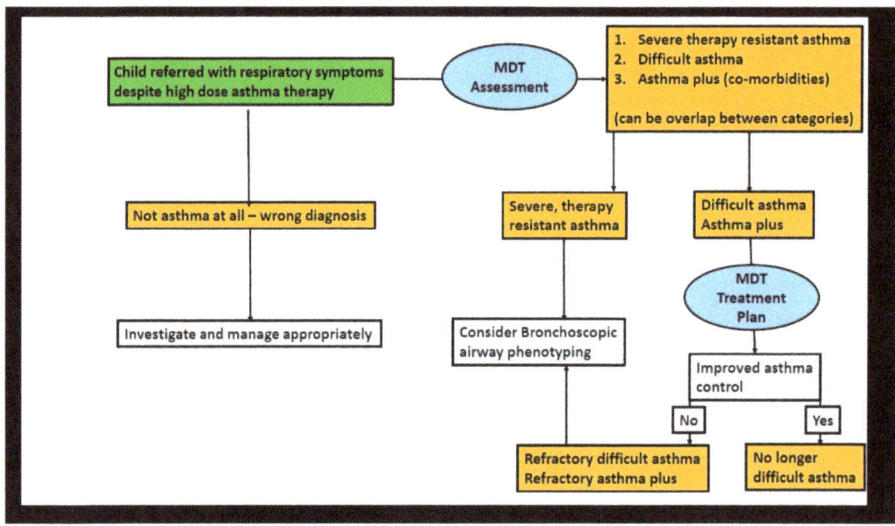

Figure 1. Flow chart for assessment of the child referred for assessment of asthma symptoms not responding to treatment. Abbreviation: MDT, multidisciplinary treatment.

The starting point is a child referred with respiratory symptoms that do not respond to asthma therapy. The first step is a detailed history and examination, with a focussed approach to testing, to exclude other diagnoses, such as vascular ring or bronchiectasis (Figure 2). The likeliest differential diagnoses will depend on geography—airway compression by tuberculous lymph nodes is rare in London, but common in high burden areas. If it is likely that the underlying diagnosis is indeed asthma, the next step is a multi-disciplinary team assessment (Table 2).

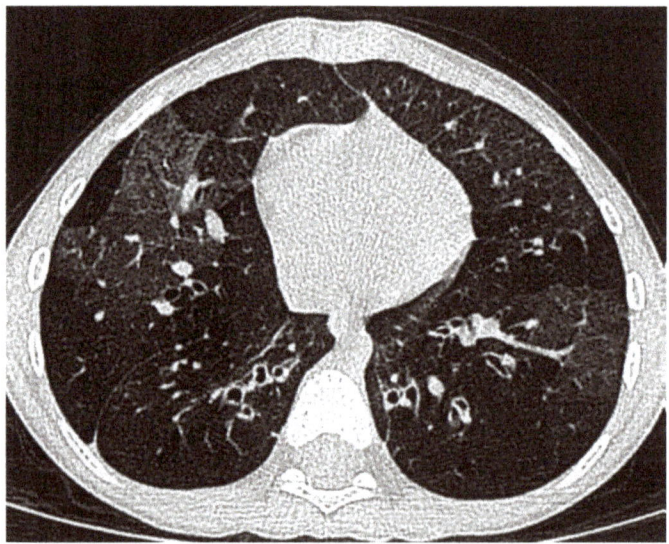

Figure 2. Not asthma at all. There is extensive large airway thickening and dilatation, with distal air trapping. This is bronchiectasis and obliterative bronchiolitis after a severe adenovirus infection.

Table 2. Multidisciplinary assessment of severe, therapy-resistant asthma.

Issue to be Addressed	Tests Performed
Symptom pattern	ACT or c-ACT, asthma attacks and prednisolone bursts, unscheduled emergency visits; evidence of severity of symptoms at emergency presentation School attendance and impact of symptoms at school
Breathing pattern disorder	Physiotherapy assessment Consider asking parents to make a video of breathing pattern Consider laryngoscopy during exercise
Psychosocial factors	Questionnaires relating to treatment burden, anxiety and depression, quality of life
Physiology	Spirometry before and after bronchodilator Lung clearance index
Allergic sensitization	Total IgE skin prick tests and specific IgE to grass and tree pollen, house dust mite, cockroach, cat and dog, aspergillus, alternaria and cladosporium and any likely relevant other antigens Not food allergens unless a suggestive clinical history
Airway inflammation	F$_E$NO Induced sputum cytospin for eosinophil count Peripheral blood eosinophil count
Nicotine exposure (tobacco or vaping, passive or active)	Urine cotinine
Medication adherence	Prescription uptake Serum prednisolone and theophylline levels if prescribed; serum inhaled corticosteroid levels if available (usually only in a research context) Electronic monitoring

Abbreviations: ACT, asthma control test; F$_E$NO = Fractional expired nitric oxide; IgE = immunoglobulin E.

There is a focus on an assessment of social and environmental factors. The child is then placed into one or more of the overlapping categories asthma plus (co-morbidities, such as obesity, food allergy, exercise-induced laryngeal obstruction (EILO [43]), rhinosinusitis), difficult asthma (asthma which could be controlled if the basics can be got right; poor adherence, adverse environmental factors such as sensitization and exposure to allergens, passive or active smoking, and psychosocial factors) and STRA. On the basis of the findings, the child with STRA goes on to invasive airway phenotyping (below), and an individualised management plan is put in place for those with difficult asthma and asthma plus. The success of the plan is reviewed two months later; many children will have responded to their plan [44], and are able to reduce treatment with improved outcomes. However, there remain a group which we term refractory asthma plus (especially obesity with failed weight loss), and refractory difficult asthma (usually continued very poor adherence or unwillingness or inability to control adverse environmental factors, such as allergen exposure) [45]. It should be remembered that poor adherence may in fact reflect STRA, and that the child and family are not taking medications which have not worked. Children with refractory asthma will also undergo invasive airway phenotyping to determine treatment. Our previous thinking was that it was not justified to give an expensive biologic to children who are not using low-dose ICS efficiently or whose parents will not get rid of an allergenic pet; we now believe that it is wrong to penalise children for the lack of adequate parenting, and we need to keep them alive despite the parenting issues. We now conclude that refractory difficult asthma due to poor adherence is not a contraindication to the use of biologicals.

The invasive phenotyping protocol is summarised in Table 3. The aim is to answer the following questions:

- Is there ongoing airway inflammation, and if so, what is the phenotype/endotype?
- Is any inflammation present steroid sensitive? (For example, corticosteroids are very effective against eosinophilic inflammation, but not in neutrophilic disease)
- Is there a disconnect between the degree of inflammation and the level of symptoms?
- Is there evidence of persistent airflow limitation?

Table 3. Invasive airway phenotyping.

Tests	First Visit	Second Visit	Third Visit
Non-invasive	Assessment of current symptoms Spirometry before and after SABA LCI F_ENO Induced sputum eosinophils	Assessment of current symptoms Spirometry before and after SABA LCI F_ENO Induced sputum eosinophils	Assessment of current symptoms Spirometry before and after SABA LCI F_ENO Induced sputum eosinophils
Invasive	Fibreoptic bronchocopy, BAL, endobronchial biopsy		
Actions	Intramuscular triamcinolone (steroid trial)	Assess steroid responsiveness Develop bespoke treatment plan	Assess response to treatment

Abbreviations: F_ENO, fractional exhaled concentration of nitric oxide; LCI, lung clearance index; SABA, short-acting beta-2 agonist.

This is particularly relevant to the obese child with asthma, who may have TH2-driven airway inflammation [46], but this is not invariable [47], and may have symptoms related to dysanaptic airway growth, defined as a normal first second forced expired volume (FEV_1), a raised forced vital capacity (FVC) and a low FEV_1/FVC ratio [48] or secondary to systemic inflammation driven by IL6 [49]. It is obviously also essential to ensure that symptoms like breathlessness are in fact not due to deconditioning [50].

If airway phenotyping has shown eosinophilic inflammation (and ideally, a transcriptomic signature for TH2 inflammation) then treatment with either omalizumab or mepolizumab may be indicated. If the phenotype is pauci-inflammatory or neutrophilic, the options are much more limited. Clearly, if the endotype is not TH2, then anti-TH2 strategies are unlikely to be successful. Options might include Tiotropium [51] or a macrolide [8], with reduction of the ICS dose [52]. However, as with adults [10], we do not have the perfect biomarker for TH2 asthma, and there may be overlapping syndromes, for example, children with neutrophilic or pauci-inflammatory disease and one or more aeroallergen sensitivities. Children with asthma may show discordance between the TH2 markers F_ENO and eosinophils, and this relationship may change over time in the same child [30]. In reality, we need to know that (for example) an IL5 endotype is driving the child's asthma before prescribing an anti-IL5 strategy, but this is not practical in current clinical practice.

It might be argued that this investigation protocol is unnecessary, and that all children with evidence of TH2-high asthma should receive a biological. However, we believe this is not a correctly focused view. Firstly, the evaluation may reveal why the asthma is severe, such as poor adherence, which at least some parents may be eager to rectify. Secondly, if we are to understand the true efficacy of biologics in children, we need to differentiate between children who have true STRA, and those for whom biologics are a fire-fighting measure to prevent the child dying. The airway endotypes in these two groups are likely to be dissimilar. Finally, given the differences between the utility of biomarkers for TH2 inflammation between children and adults, and the lack of specificity even in adults, a bronchoscopic evaluation to determine that Type 2 inflammation is actually present is fully justified to prevent the child being submitted to a long course of futile and time-consuming therapy.

7. What Are the Paediatric Data, and Who Should Get What Biologic?

There are currently five biologicals licensed in adults. These are omalizumab (binding to the high affinity IgE receptor), mepolizumab and reslizumab (both binding IL5), benralizumab (binds to IL5 receptor α subunit) and dupilumab (binds to IL4 receptor α subunit, thus blocking IL4 and IL13). Tezepilumab, which binds to TSLP, is in Phase 2B trials. Of these, only two (mepolizumab and omalizumab) are licensed for children with asthma; dupilumab is licensed for children with atopic dermatitis.

7.1. Omalizumab

Although there are fewer randomised controlled trials in children than in adults, the Cochrane review [53] was able to summarise a lot of data and give evidence-based guidelines. In summary, the suggested indications were a total IgE between 76 and 1500, evidence of aeroallergen sensitisation and multiple asthma attacks. It should be noted that around 30% of our STRA patients have a total IgE above the range of eligibility. Furthermore, adult data show that the response to omalizumab may be equally good in those meeting IgE criteria but without aeroallergen sensitization [26]. Asthma attacks are reduced by Omalizumab (odds ratio 0.55, 95% confidence intervals 0.42–0.60 in 10 studies recruiting 3261 patients). The absolute reduction in attacks was from 26% to 16%. Admissions to hospital were also decreased: odds ratio 0.16, 95% confidence intervals 0.06–0.42 in four studies recruiting 1824 patients. The absolute reduction was 3% to 0.5%. There was also a reduction in the softer end-point of short acting beta2 agonist (SABA) usage (odds ratio 0.16, 95% confidence intervals 0.06–0.42, in four studies recruiting 1824 participants). The reduction in actual use was a mean of −0.39 puffs per day, 95% confidence intervals −0.55 to −0.24 in nine studies recruiting 3524 patients.

The ERS/ATS Task Force [8] has recently suggested that a blood eosinophils ≥260/µλ and F_ENO ≥19.5 ppb are cut-offs to predict response to omalizumab in adults with severe allergic asthma, but both were conditional recommendations based on low-quality evidence (a single study [26]). There are no biomarker data sufficient to inform recommendations in younger children. The UK authorities have insisted on the need for a history of at least four attacks of asthma requiring oral corticosteroids before omalizumab can be prescribed. Given the overwhelming evidence that the best predictor of a future asthma attack and asthma deaths is a previous attack [37,54], this recommendation, which is based on "cost-effectiveness", cannot be right for children. The other restriction is that compliance to standard medications is assured. This too is wrong; firstly, because although non-adherence can be confirmed, e.g., failing to pick up or cash prescriptions or failure of activation of an electronic monitoring device [55], adherence can only be assured by directly observed therapy, which is (a) not easy to set up in clinical practice, and (b) fraught with pitfalls. Secondly, as above, children should not be allowed to die because their parents will not ensure they are taking basic treatment.

Recent data have highlighted that omalizumab may also have significant anti-viral effects. Every autumn, when the new school year begins, there is peak in asthma attacks related to respiratory viruses, and likely also worse adherence during the school summer holidays to inhaled corticosteroids. This peak of admissions was abolished in a study of more than 400 inner city children [56]. This was taken further in a study of 478 children [57]. There was a four to nine month run-in, before they were randomised before autumn 2012 and 2013 to either four months of omalizumab, or a pre-autumn boost in the prescribed dose of inhaled corticosteroids, or placebo. The biggest beneficial effect as seen in children at Step 5, and the two active treatment strategies (inhaled corticosteroid boost, omalizumab) were equally efficacious in the overall study group. However, if the child had had an asthma attack during the run-in period, omalizumab was the best strategy. In in vitro work, they demonstrated that Omalizumab boosted peripheral blood mononuclear cell IFN-α responses to rhinovirus, and this was correlated with clinical response. The authors therefore recommended the use of omalizumab only in those children having asthma attacks despite step 5 therapy.

7.2. Mepolizumab

The ERS/ATS Task Force [8] has made recommendations for the use of the anti-IL5 monoclonal mepolizumab. They suggested that mepolizumab should be used in adults as add-on therapy for patients with severe uncontrolled asthma with an eosinophilic phenotype. This was a conditional recommendation based on, at best, moderate quality of evidence. Mepolizumab reduced asthma attacks and hospitalizations and led to reduction in dose in those prescribed maintenance oral corticosteroid. The effects on asthma control, quality of life and FEV_1 did not achieve the minimal clinically important difference.

Drug-related adverse events were slightly higher in those assigned to mepolizumab. Disappointingly, although an entry criterion for the mepolizumab trials was an age of 12 years and older, there were only 34 participants who were not adults. In the 6–11 year age group, the data are largely safety and pharmacokinetic [18] with only minimal efficacy data. Enrolment for these studies was on standard adult criteria, namely blood eosinophils ≥300/μλ at screening or ≥150/μλ in the previous year, and the dose was 40mg if body weight <40kg, 100mg if >40kg. It was unclear how many children met the ERS/ATS definition of STRA [36]. Studied end-points were adverse events, blood eosinophil counts, annualised exacerbation rate and asthma control (ACQ/c-ACT). Less than 50 children have been studied in total, for a total of one year. The overall conclusions were that no new safety issues were raised, and there was a marked decline in peripheral blood eosinophil counts, similar to those seen in adults. Such conclusions on efficacy as could be drawn were promising, but further work is needed. However, despite the paucity of data in young children, mepolizumab has been approved in children age six and over by EMA (European Medicines Agency). A trial of mepolizumab is of course reasonable in children age six and over who meet the blood eosinophil criteria and are having attacks if they fail to respond to omalizumab or are not eligible because the IgE is too high, but the paediatrician should remain aware of the limitations of the efficacy data of this biologic.

Another potential role for mepolizumab, not studied at all in children, is as adjunctive therapy after an asthma attack. The UK National Review of Asthma Deaths (NRAD) has taught us that the month after an attack is the period of highest risk for asthma deaths [37]; and we know that uncontrolled Type 2 inflammation is also a risk factor. Hence, we need a trial to determine whether a single dose of mepolizumab before the child is discharged from hospital after a severe attack could improve outcomes.

8. Limitations of Current Clinical Trials

As highlighted above, there is a paucity of studies in children, and even those studies which recruited children over the age of 12, in practice recruited adults almost exclusively. This must not be allowed to continue. Trials have assumed that biomarkers which are important in adults are correct for children, but this may not be the case. They have assumed that the safety issues are the same in children and adults. We are doing our children a disservice by uncritically extrapolating from adults to children. We need an international collaboration to recruit large numbers of carefully characterised children, with a wide range of biomarkers prospectively measured so we can learn how to predict responders in the future. We also need studies comparing the biologics in children.

9. Summary and Conclusions: Where from Here?

It is clear that there are important differences between paediatric and adult STRA. Paediatric STRA is often eosinophilic, but frequently, there is no evidence that the TH2 pathway is in play. There are significant doubts that peripheral blood eosinophil count relate closely to eosinophilic airway inflammation; eosinophilic inflammation may not be TH2 driven, at least in many cases; sputum cellular phenotype may not be consistent over time, and the eosinophil may have developmental roles which mean that anti-eosinophil strategies may have unanticipated consequences in young children. It is therefore clear that extrapolating adult data into the paediatric age group is potentially hazardous. The inescapable conclusion is that we need trials in children, and the regulatory authorities need to hold Pharma to account to ensure these studies are done.

The prerequisites for such studies include the careful characterisation of the patients; are they asthmatics who could be controlled on low-dose ICS if they were used properly, and thus it is likely the TH2 endotype is relevant, or are they true STRA, in which case, multiple different endotypes are probably important? The first pressing need is to determine who should be prescribed omalizumab and who mepolizumab, as these are the two biologicals licensed for children. A high proportion of

STRA children may be eligible for either, and we have no current means of determining the best course of action. At the moment, in such cases, most would start with omalizumab as the biological with which we have the most experience. A head-to-head comparison trial is urgently needed, and is shortly commencing in the UK [58]. However, there are an increasing number of biologicals relevant to the TH2 pathway which will also become licensed in children, and we urgently need biomarkers to enable us to choose between them on a rational basis, rather than doing a succession of N-of-1 trials, with all the issues of placebo effects. Furthermore, perhaps combinations may be better—for example, mepolizumab (anti-IL5) and dupilumab (anti-IL4/IL13) co-administered might be a better anti-TH2 strategy than either alone, but this must be tested. This also highlights that we need objective biomarkers of response; clearly, if a child with an attack-prone phenotype is started on biological and ceases to have attacks, the benefits are clear-cut, but some benefits are less objective.

Another real challenge to the paediatric respiratory community is the anti-Il13 (trakilizumab) story. This agent was (ethically correctly) studied in adults and was found to be ineffective, and discarded [59]. Given the differences outlined above between adult and paediatric STRA, is it conceivable that trakilizumab could be effective in children but not in adults? And how could we ethically do such studies in children? There may be two possible answers. The first is assessing the effects in developmentally appropriate, physiological models of asthma, such as the murine neonatal, house dust mite inhalational challenge model, which recapitulates the features of early onset allergic airways disease [60]. The second may be to define biomarkers for a subgroup of IL13 upregulated patients—conceivably those with high F_ENO and low sputum eosinophil counts.

A further, as yet unsolved, challenge is how to halt the march from pre-school viral wheeze, with no evidence of TH2 inflammation, to atopic, school-age asthma [61]. We know from three definitive randomised controlled trials that an early use of inhaled corticosteroids is not the answer [62–64]. Could an early institution of therapy be directed more specifically at TH2 inflammation, such as mepolizumab? For this to be explored, we need better to understand the endotypes, and especially find biomarkers to predict those who are at risk of disease evolution; current predictive indices have a high negative predictive value, but their positive predictive value is much less useful [65,66].

In summary, the advent of the new biological agents have brought us to the edge of a new age in asthma management. If the benefits are to be realised, we must insist that clinical trials are performed in children, and specifically that regulatory authorities insist on the submission of a credible paediatric investigation plan as a condition of permitting adult studies to be done. We need to get cleverer, abandoning umbrella terms like asthma, and determining endotypes in a way that is practical in the clinic. In this way, we can match the child to the most appropriate treatment. However, the final word in all asthma manuscripts like this must be that most children do not need expensive novel therapies to control their asthma. If the basics are got right, and low-dose ICS are used regularly and correctly, then most asthma becomes a disease that is eminently treatable.

Conflicts of Interest: The author declare no conflict of interest.

References

1. Pavord, I.D.; Beasley, R.; Agusti, A.; Anderson, G.P.; Bel, E.; Brusselle, G.; Frey, U. After asthma—redefining airways diseases. *Lancet* **2018**, *391*, 350–400. [CrossRef]
2. Brown, H.M. Treatment of chronic asthma with prednisolone; significance of eosinophils in the sputum. *Lancet* **1958**, *2*, 1245–1247. [CrossRef]
3. Leckie, M.J.; ten Brinke, A.; Khan, J.; Diamant, Z.; O'Connor, B.J.; Walls, C.M.; Hansel, T.T. Effects of an interleukin-5 Blocking Monoclonal Antibody on Eosinophils, Airway Hyper-Responsiveness, and the Late Asthmatic Response. *Lancet* **2000**, *356*, 2144–2148. [CrossRef]
4. Nair, P.; Pizzichini, M.M.; Kjarsgaard, M.; Inman, M.D.; Efthimiadis, A.; Pizzichini, E.; O'Byrne, P.M. Mepolizumab for Prednisone-Dependent Asthma with Sputum Eosinophilia. *N. Engl. J. Med.* **2009**, *360*, 985–993. [CrossRef]

5. Haldar, P.; Brightling, C.E.; Hargadon, B.; Gupta, S.; Monteiro, W.; Sousa, A.; Pavord, I.D. Mepolizumab and exacerbations of refractory eosinophilic asthma. *N. Engl. J. Med.* **2009**, *360*, 973–984. [CrossRef]
6. De Boeck, K.; Amaral, M.D. Progress in Therapies for Cystic Fibrosis. *Lancet Respir. Med.* **2016**, *4*, 662–674. [CrossRef]
7. Ramsey, B.W.; Davies, J.; McElvaney, N.G.; Tullis, E.; Bell, S.C.; Dřevínek, P.; Moss, R. VX08-770-102 Study Group. A CFTR Potentiator in Patients with Cystic Fibrosis and the G551D Mutation. *N. Engl. J. Med.* **2011**, *365*, 1663–1672. [CrossRef] [PubMed]
8. Holguin, F.; Cardet, J.C.; Chung, K.F.; Diver, S.; Ferreira, D.S.; Fitzpatrick, A.; Gaga, M.; Kellermeyer, L.; Khurana, S.; Knight, S.; et al. Management of Severe Asthma: A European Respiratory Society/American Thoracic Society Guideline. *Eur. Respir. J.* **2019**, *26*, 1900588. [CrossRef]
9. Pavord, I.D.; Korn, S.; Howarth, P.; Bleecker, E.R.; Buhl, R.; Keene, O.N.; Chanez, P. Mepolizumab for severe eosinophilic asthma (DREAM): A multicentre, double-blind, placebo-controlled trial. *Lancet* **2012**, *380*, 651–659. [CrossRef]
10. Pavlidis, S.; Takahashi, K.; Kwong, F.N.K.; Xie, J.; Hoda, U.; Sun, K.; Chanez, P. "T2-high" in severe asthma related to blood eosinophil, exhaled nitric oxide and serum periostin. *Eur. Respir. J.* **2018**, *53*, 1800938. [CrossRef] [PubMed]
11. Kuo, C.H.S.; Pavlidis, S.; Loza, M.; Baribaud, F.; Rowe, A.; Pandis, I.; Sterk, P.J. T-helper Cell Type 2 (Th2) and non-Th2 Molecular Phenotypes of Asthma Using Sputum Transcriptomics in U-BIOPRED. *Eur. Respir. J.* **2017**, *49*, 28179442. [CrossRef] [PubMed]
12. Wang, H.B.; Weller, P.F. Pivotal advance: Eosinophils mediate early alum adjuvant-elicited B cell priming and IgM production. *J. Leukoc. Biol.* **2008**, *83*, 817–821. [CrossRef] [PubMed]
13. Fröhlich, A.; Steinhauser, G.; Scheel, T.; Roch, T.; Fillatreau, S.; Lee, J.J.; Berek, C. Eosinophils are required for the maintenance of plasma cells in the bone marrow. *Nat. Immunol.* **2011**, *12*, 151–159.
14. Xenakis, J.J.; Howard, E.D.; Smith, K.M.; Olbrich, C.L.; Huang, Y.; Anketell, D.; Spencer, L.A. Resident intestinal eosinophils constitutively express antigen presentation markers and include two phenotypically distinct subsets of eosinophils. *Immunology* **2018**, *154*, 298–308. [CrossRef] [PubMed]
15. Wu, D.; Molofsky, A.B.; Liang, H.E.; Ricardo-Gonzalez, R.R.; Jouihan, H.A.; Bando, J.K.; Locksley, R.M. Eosinophils sustain adipose alternatively activated macrophages associated with glucose homeostasis. *Science* **2011**, *332*, 243–247. [CrossRef]
16. Qiu, Y.; Nguyen, K.D.; Odegaard, J.I.; Cui, X.; Tian, X.; Locksley, R.M.; Chawla, A. Eosinophils and type 2 cytokine signaling in macrophages orchestrate development of functional beige fat. *Cell* **2014**, *157*, 1292–1308. [CrossRef]
17. Sabogal Piñeros, Y.S.; Bal, S.M.; Dijkhuis, A.; Majoor, C.J.; Dierdorp, B.S.; Dekker, T.; Koenderman, L. Eosinophils Capture Viruses, a Capacity That Is Defective in Asthma. *Allergy* **2019**, *74*, 1898–1909. [CrossRef]
18. Gupta, A.; Ikeda, M.; Geng, B.; Azmi, J.; Price, R.G.; Bradford, E.S.; Yancey, S.W.; Steinfeld, J. Long-term Safety and Pharmacodynamics of Mepolizumab in Children with Severe Asthma With an Eosinophilic Phenotype. *J. Allergy Clin. Immunol.* **2019**, *144*, 1336–1342. [CrossRef]
19. Saglani, S.; Lui, S.; Ullmann, N.; Campbell, G.A.; Sherburn, R.T.; Mathie, S.A.; Denney, L.; Bossley, C.J.; Oates, T.; Walker, S.A.; et al. IL-33 promotes airway remodeling in pediatric patients with severe, steroid-resistant asthma. *J. Allergy Clin. Immunol.* **2013**, *132*, 676–685. [CrossRef]
20. Castanhinha, S.; Sherburn, R.; Walker, S.; Gupta, A.; Bossley, C.J.; Buckley, J.; Ullmann, N.; Grychtol, R.; Campbell, G.; Maglione, M.; et al. Pediatric severe asthma with fungal sensitization is mediated by steroid-resistant IL-33. *J. Allergy Clin. Immunol.* **2015**, *136*, 312–322. [CrossRef]
21. Fitzpatrick, A.M. National Institutes of Health/National Heart, Lung and Blood Institute's Severe Asthma Research Program. The molecular phenotype of severe asthma in children. *J. Allergy Clin. Immunol.* **2010**, *125*, 851–857. [CrossRef] [PubMed]
22. Wisniewski, J.A.; Muehling, L.M.; Eccles, J.D.; Capaldo, B.J.; Agrawal, R.; Shirley, D.A.; Teague, W.G. T_H1 signatures are present in the lower airways of children with severe asthma, regardless of allergic status. *J. Allergy Clin. Immunol.* **2018**, *141*, 2048–2060. [CrossRef] [PubMed]
23. Fleming, L.; Tsartsali, L.; Wilson, N.; Regamey, N.; Bush, A. Sputum inflammatory phenotypes are not stable in children with asthma. *Thorax* **2012**, *67*, 675–681. [CrossRef] [PubMed]
24. Wark, P.A.B.; Simpson, J.; Hensley, M.J.; Gibson, P.G. Airway Inflammation in Thunderstorm Asthma. *Clin. Exp. Allergy* **2002**, *32*, 1750–1756. [CrossRef] [PubMed]

25. Petsky, H.L.; Cates, C.J.; Kew, K.M.; Chang, A.B. Tailoring Asthma Treatment on Eosinophilic Markers (Exhaled Nitric Oxide or Sputum Eosinophils): A Systematic Review and Meta-Analysis. *Thorax* **2018**, *73*, 1110–1119. [CrossRef]
26. Van den Berge, M.; Pauw, R.G.; de Monchy, J.G.; van Minnen, C.A.; Postma, D.S.; Kerstjens, H.A. Beneficial effects of treatment with anti-IgE antibodies (Omalizumab) in a patient with severe asthma and negative skin-prick test results. *Chest* **2011**, *139*, 190–193. [CrossRef]
27. Fitzpatrick, A.M.; Jackson, D.J.; Mauger, D.T.; Boehmer, S.J.; Phipatanakul, W.; Sheehan, W.J.; Covar, R. NIH/NHLBI AsthmaNet. Individualized Therapy for Persistent Asthma in Young Children. *J. Allergy Clin. Immunol.* **2016**, *138*, 1608–1618.e12. [CrossRef]
28. Ullmann, N.; Bossley, C.J.; Fleming, L.; Silvestri, M.; Bush, A.; Saglani, S. Blood eosinophil counts rarely reflect airway eosinophilia in children with severe asthma. *Allergy* **2013**, *68*, 402–406. [CrossRef]
29. Fleming, L.; Koo, M.; Bossley, C.J.; Nagakumar, P.; Bush, A.; Saglani, S. The utility of a multidomain assessment of steroid response for predicting clinical response to omalizumab. *J. Allergy Clin. Immunol.* **2016**, *138*, 292–294. [CrossRef]
30. Fleming, L.; Tsartsali, L.; Wilson, N.; Regamey, N.; Bush, A. Longitudinal Relationship between Sputum Eosinophils and Exhaled Nitric Oxide in Children with Asthma. *Am. J. Respir. Crit. Care Med.* **2013**, *188*, 400–402. [CrossRef]
31. Shrimanker, R.; Keene, O.; Hynes, G.; Wenzel, S.; Yancey, S.; Pavord, I.D. Prognostic and predictive value of blood eosinophil count, fractional exhaled nitric oxide, and their combination in severe asthma: A *post hoc* analysis. *Am. J. Respir. Crit. Care Med.* **2019**, *200*, 1308–1311. [CrossRef] [PubMed]
32. Bracken, M.B.; Fleming, L.; Hall, P.; Van Stiphout, N.; Bossley, C.J.; Biggart, E.; Wilson, N.M.; Bush, A. The importance of nurse led home visits in the assessment of children with problematic asthma. *Arch. Dis. Child* **2009**, *94*, 780–784. [CrossRef] [PubMed]
33. Strunk, R.C.; Bacharier, L.B.; Phillips, B.R.; Szefler, S.J.; Zeiger, R.S.; Chinchilli, V.M.; Morgan, W.J. CARE Network. Azithromycin or montelukast as inhaled corticosteroid-sparing agents in moderate-to-severe childhood asthma study. *J. Allergy Clin. Immunol.* **2008**, *122*, 1138–1144. [CrossRef] [PubMed]
34. Szefler, S.J.; Mitchell, H.; Sorkness, C.A.; Gergen, P.J.; T O'Connor, G.; Morgan, W.J.; Eggleston, P.A. Management of asthma based on exhaled nitric oxide in addition to guideline-based treatment for inner-city adolescents and young adults: A randomised controlled trial. *Lancet* **2008**, *372*, 1065–1072. [CrossRef]
35. Lemanske, R.F., Jr.; Mauger, D.T.; Sorkness, C.A.; Jackson, D.J.; Boehmer, S.J.; Martinez, F.D.; Covar, R.A. Childhood Asthma Research and Education (CARE) Network of the National Heart, Lung, and Blood Institute. Step-up therapy for children with uncontrolled asthma receiving inhaled corticosteroids. *N. Engl. J. Med.* **2010**, *362*, 975–985. [CrossRef]
36. Chung, K.F.; Wenzel, S.E.; Brozek, J.L.; Bush, A.; Castro, M.; Sterk, P.J.; Adcock, I.M.; Bateman, E.D.; Bel, E.H.; Bleecker, E.R.; et al. International ERS/ATS guidelines on definition, evaluation and treatment of severe asthma. *Eur. Respir. J.* **2014**, *43*, 343–373. [CrossRef]
37. Available online: https://www.rcplondon.ac.uk/file/868/download?token=JQzyNWUs (accessed on 23 April 2020).
38. Suissa, S.; Ernst, P.; Boivin, J.F.; Horwitz, R.I.; Habbick, B.; Cockroft, D.; Blais, L.; McNutt, M.; Buist, A.S.; Spitzer, W.O. A cohort analysis of excess mortality in asthma and the use of inhaled beta-agonists. *Am. J. Respir. Crit. Care Med.* **1994**, *149*, 604–610. [CrossRef]
39. Spitzer, W.O.; Suissa, S.; Ernst, P.; Horwitz, R.I.; Habbick, B.; Cockcroft, D.; Rebuck, A.S. The use of β-agonists and the risk of death and near death from asthma. *N. Engl. J. Med.* **1992**, *326*, 501–506. [CrossRef]
40. Bush, A.; Saglani, S. Management of severe asthma in children. *Lancet* **2010**, *376*, 814–825. [CrossRef]
41. Cook, J.; Beresford, F.; Fainardi, V.; Hall, P.; Housley, G.; Jamalzadeh, A.; Nightingale, M.; Winch, D.; Bush, A.; Fleming, L.; et al. Managing the paediatric patient with refractory asthma: A multidisciplinary approach. *J. Asthma Allergy* **2017**, *10*, 123–130. [CrossRef]
42. Bush, A.; Fleming, L.; Saglani, S. Severe asthma in children. *Respirology* **2017**, *22*, 886–897. [CrossRef] [PubMed]
43. Halvorsen, T.; Walsted, E.S.; Bucca, C.; Bush, A.; Cantarella, G.; Friedrich, G.; Herth, F.J.F.; Hull, J.H.; Jung, H.; Maat, R.; et al. Inducible laryngeal obstruction: An official joint European Respiratory Society and European Laryngological Society statement. *Eur. Respir. J.* **2017**, *50*, 1602221. [CrossRef] [PubMed]

44. Sharples, J.; Gupta, A.; Fleming, L.; Bossley, C.J.; Bracken-King, M.; Hall, P.; Hayward, A.; Puckey, M.; Balfour-Lynn, I.M.; Rosenthal, M.; et al. Long-term effectiveness of a staged assessment for paediatric problematic severe asthma [Research Letter]. *Eur. Respir. J.* **2012**, *40*, 264–267. [CrossRef] [PubMed]
45. Bush, A.; Saglani, S.; Fleming, L. Severe asthma: Looking beyond the amount of medication. *Lancet Respir. Med.* **2017**, *5*, 844–846. [CrossRef]
46. Desai, D.; Newby, C.; Symon, F.A.; Haldar, P.; Shah, S.; Gupta, S.; Herath, A. Elevated sputum interleukin-5 and submucosal eosinophilia in obese individuals with severe asthma. *Am. J. Respir. Crit. Care Med.* **2013**, *188*, 657–663. [CrossRef] [PubMed]
47. Van Huisstede, A.; Rudolphus, A.; van Schadewijk, A.; Cabezas, M.C.; Mannaerts, G.H.; Taube, C.; Braunstahl, G.J. Bronchial and systemic inflammation in morbidly obese subjects with asthma: A biopsy study. *Am. J. Respir. Crit. Care Med.* **2014**, *190*, 951–954. [CrossRef] [PubMed]
48. Forno, E.; Weiner, D.J.; Mullen, J.; Sawicki, G.; Kurland, G.; Han, Y.Y.; Cloutier, M.M.; Canino, G.; Weiss, S.T.; Litonjua, A.A.; et al. Obesity and Airway Dysanapsis in Children with and without Asthma. *Am. J. Respir. Crit. Care Med.* **2017**, *195*, 314–323. [CrossRef] [PubMed]
49. Peters, M.C.; McGrath, K.W.; Hawkins, G.A.; Hastie, A.T.; Levy, B.D.; Israel, E.; Johansson, M.W. National Heart, Lung, and Blood Institute Severe Asthma Research Program. Plasma interleukin-6 concentrations, metabolic dysfunction, and asthma severity: A cross-sectional analysis of two cohorts. *Lancet Respir. Med.* **2016**, *4*, 574–584. [CrossRef]
50. Johansson, H.; Norlander, K.; Berglund, L.; Janson, C.; Malinovschi, A.; Nordvall, L.; Emtner, M. Prevalence of exercise-induced bronchoconstriction and exercise-induced laryngeal obstruction in a general adolescent population. *Thorax* **2015**, *70*, 57–63. [CrossRef]
51. Vogelberg, C.; Szefler, S.J.; Vrijlandt, E.J.; Boner, A.L.; Engel, M.; El Azzi, G.; Hamelmann, E.H. Tiotropium add-on therapy is safe and reduces seasonal worsening in paediatric asthma patients. *Eur. Respir. J.* **2019**, *53*, 31097514. [CrossRef]
52. Lazarus, S.C.; Krishnan, J.A.; King, T.S.; Lang, J.E.; Blake, K.V.; Covar, R.; Dyer, A.M. National Heart, Lung, and Blood Institute AsthmaNet. Mometasone or Tiotropium in Mild Asthma with a Low Sputum Eosinophil Level. *N. Engl. J. Med.* **2019**, *380*, 2009–2019. [CrossRef] [PubMed]
53. Normansell, R.; Walker, S.; Milan, S.J.; Walters, E.H.; Nair, P. Omalizumab for asthma in adults and children. *Cochrane Database Syst. Rev.* **2014**, *1*, CD003559. [CrossRef] [PubMed]
54. Buelo, A.; McLean, S.; Julious, S.; Flores-Kim, J.; Bush, A.; Henderson, J.; Paton, J.Y.; Sheikh, A.; Shields, M.; Pinnock, H. At-risk children with asthma (ARC): A systematic review. *Thorax* **2018**, *73*, 813–824. [CrossRef] [PubMed]
55. Jochmann, A.; Artusio, L.; Jamalzadeh, A.; Nagakumar, P.; Delgado-Eckert, E.; Saglani, S.; Bush, A.; Frey, U.; Fleming, L. Electronic monitoring of adherence to inhaled corticosteroids: An essential tool in identifying severe asthma in children. *Eur. Respir. J.* **2017**, *50*, 1700910. [CrossRef]
56. Busse, W.W.; Morgan, W.J.; Gergen, P.J.; Mitchell, H.E.; Gern, J.E.; Liu, A.H.; Gruchalla, R.S.; Kattan, M.; Teach, S.J.; Pongracic, J.A.; et al. Randomized trial of omalizumab (anti-IgE) for asthma in inner-city children. *N. Engl. J. Med.* **2011**, *364*, 1005–1015. [CrossRef]
57. Teach, S.J.; Gill, M.A.; Togias, A.; Sorkness, C.A.; Arbes, S.J., Jr.; Calatroni, A.; Kercsmar, C.M. Preseasonal Treatment with Either Omalizumab or an Inhaled Corticosteroid Boost to Prevent Fall Asthma Exacerbations. *J. Allergy Clin. Immunol.* **2015**, *136*, 1476–1485. [CrossRef]
58. Saglani, S.; Bush, A.; Carroll, W.; Cunningham, S.; Fleming, L.; Gaillard, E.; Roberts, G. Biologics for paediatric severe asthma: Trick or TREAT. *Lancet Respir. Med.* **2019**, *7*, 294–296. [CrossRef]
59. Russell, R.J.; Chachi, L.; FitzGerald, J.M.; Backer, V.; Olivenstein, R.; Titlestad, I.L.; Leaker, B. MESOS study investigators. Effect of Tralokinumab, an interleukin-13 Neutralising Monoclonal Antibody, on Eosinophilic Airway Inflammation in Uncontrolled Moderate-To-Severe Asthma (MESOS): A Multicentre, Double-Blind, Randomised, Placebo-Controlled Phase 2 Trial. *Lancet Respir. Med.* **2018**, *6*, 499–510.
60. Saglani, S.; Mathie, S.A.; Gregory, L.G.; Bell, M.J.; Bush, A.; Lloyd, C.M. Pathophysiological Features of Asthma Develop in Parallel in House Dust Mite Exposed Neonatal Mice. *Am. J. Respir. Cell Mol. Biol.* **2009**, *41*, 281–289. [CrossRef]

61. Turner, S.; Custovic, A.; Ghazal, P.; Grigg, J.; Gore, M.; Henderson, J.; Lloyd, C.M.; Marsland, B.; Power, U.F.; Roberts, G.; et al. Pulmonary epithelial barrier and immunological functions at birth and in early life - key determinants of the development of asthma? A description of the protocol for the Breathing Together study. *Wellcome Open Res.* **2018**, *3*, 60. [CrossRef]
62. Guilbert, T.W.; Morgan, W.J.; Zeiger, R.S.; Mauger, D.T.; Boehmer, S.J.; Szefler, S.J.; Bloomberg, G.R. Long-term inhaled corticosteroids in preschool children at high risk for asthma. *N. Engl. J. Med.* **2006**, *354*, 1985–1997. [CrossRef] [PubMed]
63. Murray, C.S.; Woodcock, A.; Langley, S.J.; Morris, J.; Custovic, A. Secondary prevention of asthma by the use of Inhaled Fluticasone propionate in Wheezy INfants (IFWIN): Double-blind, randomised, controlled study. *Lancet* **2006**, *368*, 754–762. [CrossRef]
64. Bisgaard, H.; Hermansen, M.N.; Loland, L.; Halkjaer, L.B.; Buchvald, F. Intermittent inhaled corticosteroids in infants with episodic wheezing. *N. Engl. J. Med.* **2006**, *354*, 1998–2005. [CrossRef] [PubMed]
65. Guilbert, T.W.; Morgan, W.J.; Krawiec, M.; Lemanske, R.F., Jr.; Sorkness, C.; Szefler, S.J.; Strunk, R.C. The Prevention of Early Asthma in Kids study: Design, rationale and methods for the Childhood Asthma Research and Education network. *Control. Clin. Trials* **2004**, *25*, 286–310. [CrossRef]
66. Devulapalli, C.S.; Carlsen, K.C.L.; Håland, G.; Munthe-Kaas, M.C.; Pettersen, M.; Mowinckel, P.; Carlsen, K.H. Severity of Obstructive Airways Disease by Age 2 Years Predicts Asthma at 10 Years of Age. *Thorax* **2008**, *63*, 8–13. [CrossRef]

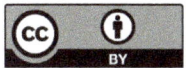 © 2020 by the author. Licensee MDPI, Basel, Switzerland. This article is an open access article distributed under the terms and conditions of the Creative Commons Attribution (CC BY) license (http://creativecommons.org/licenses/by/4.0/).

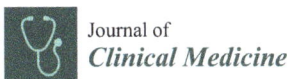

Article

Asthma-Like Features and Anti-Asthmatic Drug Prescription in Children with Non-CF Bronchiectasis

Konstantinos Douros [1], Olympia Sardeli [1], Spyridon Prountzos [2], Angeliki Galani [1], Dafni Moriki [1], Efthymia Alexopoulou [2] and Kostas N. Priftis [1,*]

[1] Allergology and Pulmonology Unit, 3rd Paediatric Department, National and Kapodistrian University of Athens, 12462 Athens, Greece; costasdouros@gmail.com (K.D.); ol.sardeli@googlemail.com (O.S.); angeliki.galani@gmail.com (A.G.); dafnimoriki@yahoo.gr (D.M.)

[2] 2nd Radiology Department, National and Kapodistrian University of Athens, Attikon University Hospital, 12462 Athens, Greece; spyttt@gmail.com (S.P.); ealex64@hotmail.com (E.A.)

* Correspondence: kpriftis@otenet.gr

Received: 15 November 2020; Accepted: 8 December 2020; Published: 11 December 2020

Abstract: Bronchiectasis and asthma may share some characteristics and some patients may have both conditions. The present study aimed to examine the rationale of prophylactic inhaled corticosteroids (ICS) prescription in children with bronchiectasis. Data of children with radiologically established bronchiectasis were retrospectively reviewed. Episodes of dyspnea and wheezing, spirometric indices, total serum IgE, blood eosinophil counts, sensitization to aeroallergens, and air-trapping on expiratory CT scans, were recorded. The study included 65 children 1.5–16 years old, with non-CF bronchiectasis. Episodes of dyspnea or wheezing were reported by 22 (33.8%) and 23 (35.4%), respectively. Skin prick tests to aeroallergens (SPTs) were positive in 15 (23.0%) patients. Mosaic pattern on CT scans was observed in 37 (56.9%) patients. Dyspnea, presence of mosaic pattern, positive reversibility test, and positive SPTs were significantly correlated with the prescription of ICS. The prescription of ICS in children with bronchiectasis is more likely when there are certain asthma-like characteristics. The difficulty to set the diagnosis of real asthma in cases of bronchiectasis may justify the decision of clinicians to start an empirical trial with ICS in certain cases.

Keywords: inhaled corticosteroids; non-CF bronchiectasis; asthma; children

1. Introduction

Bronchiectasis is a complex and progressive respiratory disorder, characterized by chronic infection, inflammation, and abnormal dilatation of the bronchi. The loss of bronchial wall integrity, the mucus impaction and mucosal oedema may reduce the lumen opening and restrict the airflow especially during expiration when the bronchial walls appose. Bronchiectasis is a syndrome and not a disease per se, and several causative and associated disorders have been described [1].

Children with bronchiectasis, apart from cough, may also develop wheeze and asthma symptoms. with reported rates ranging from 11 to 46% [2,3], although it is not always clear if this is a consequence of coexistent asthma, or is a direct result of bronchiectasis. The difficulty in clarifying this point is not only due to the scarcity of adequate data but also to the lack of a simple clinical tool to identify asthma in children and, the vagueness of the main clinical characteristics of asthma. Indeed, dyspnea is a subjective feeling of the patient [4] and wheezing can be easily confused with other respiratory sounds especially when its presence is reported by patients or parents [5]. However, there is no doubt that asthma and bronchiectasis do coexist in some patients, and despite the absence of clear information on a mechanism linking the two conditions, the apparent implication of their overlap is a more severe disease with more frequent exacerbations [6].

The treatment of bronchiectasis is based mainly on antibiotics and chest physiotherapy. In cases of bronchiectasis and asthma coexistence, patients must receive treatment for both conditions [7,8]. Nevertheless, in daily practice, inhaled corticosteroids, with or without long-acting beta-agonists (LABA), are frequently prescribed in patients with bronchiectasis even when there is no clear evidence of coexisting asthma. Although the reason that drives physicians to adopt this non-evidence based practice is not clear, it might be related to the limited treatment options, the variable and often non-satisfactory response to therapy, and the frequent exacerbations of bronchiectasis. The present study aimed to describe the extent of the empirical use of ICS in children with bronchiectasis and the rationale behind the implementation of this practice.

2. Methods

The present study was conducted in the Pediatric Pulmonology Unit of the Attikon University Hospital in Athens, which is one of the main tertiary referral centres for pediatric pulmonary disorders, in Greece. Three consultants and four fellows had been serving in the Unit during the study period. Data of all the children attended in the Unit from 2013 to 2018, up to 16 years old, with chronic wet cough and radiologically established bronchiectasis on chest high-resolution computed tomography (HRCT) scan were retrospectively reviewed. All HRCT scans had been performed in the radiology department of our hospital and were evaluated by the same pediatric radiologist who was aware of the patients' clinical history. The criteria for the diagnosis of bronchiectasis on HRCT were dilatation of bronchi, as determined by broncho-arterial ratio > 0.80 [8,9]; parallel bronchial walls in a longitudinal section (tram sign); visualization of bronchi within 1 cm of pleura. We used the modified Bhalla score to quantify the severity of bronchiectasis [10]. The presence of areas of decreased attenuation on expiration ("mosaic attenuation") suggestive of airways obstruction was recorded.

Investigations in all patients included a complete blood count, sweat test and/or cystic fibrosis (CF) gene mutation analysis, measurement of serum immunoglobulins, and skin prick tests (SPT) to the most common aeroallergens (olive, grass, Parietaria, Chenopodium, cypress, house dust mite, fungi, cat and dog dander). Nasal nitric oxide test and high-speed video microscopy analysis were performed only in patients who fit the clinical phenotype of primary ciliary dyskinesia. Spirometry was performed at the initial and the follow-up visits to all patients ≥5 years old who were able to cooperate. T_H2-high status was defined as the combination of total serum IgE levels of ≥100 IU/mL and absolute blood eosinophil count of ≥140/mL [11].

All patients who reported episodes of dyspnea (shortness of breath) or wheezing, and/or their spirometric indices or the shape of the spirometry loop were indicative of airway obstruction, and/or had positive SPT, underwent a bronchodilator response (BDR) test with salbutamol, during their first visit. The BDR test was performed with four actuations of salbutamol metered dose inhaler into a spacer device and interpreted as positive if the change in the forced expiratory volume in one second (FEV1) after bronchodilator administration was ≥ 12%. Spirometric indices were reported as percent predicted (pp) values using the NHANES III reference equations. All patients received antibiotics for 3–6 weeks, started daily chest physiotherapy, and some of them were also prescribed ICS with or without LABA. All were reevaluated in 2–3 months.

Patients with CF were excluded from the study.

The study protocol was approved by the Attikon University Hospital Ethics Committee.

Statistical Analysis

Variables are presented as mean with standard deviation (sd) or as median with interquartile range (IQR). Univariate analysis was performed with paired t-test, chi-square test, and Spearman's rank correlation test with Bonferroni correction for multiple comparisons. Correlations were expressed as Spearman's ρ with its corresponding 95% confidence interval (CI). The variables which in univariate analysis were significantly correlated with the decision to start ICS were included as explanatory variables in a multivariate logistic regression model. Results of multivariate analysis are presented as odds ratios (OR) with 95% confidence interval (CI). We further performed three linear regression models where ICS use was the explanatory variable and the differences in FEV1, FEV1/FVC, and the number of positive cultures, between the follow-up and the initial visit, were used as the response variables.

3. Results

Sixty-five children 1.5–16 years old, were diagnosed with non-CF bronchiectasis; 46 (70.7%) of them had been referred as cases of difficult asthma. Thirty-nine (60%) children had been referred by general pediatric practitioners, and 26 (40%) by pediatric departments and clinics. Sixteen (24.6%) patients had underlying disorders directly or possibly related with bronchiectasis: five had tracheoesophageal atresia, five had PCD, one had Crohn disease that was treated with infliximab, one had Job syndrome, one had congenital pulmonary airway malformation (CPAM), one had anhidrotic ectodermal dysplasia with immunodeficiency, and one had IgA deficiency. The remaining 49 (75.4%) patients had no identifiable cause. Apart from the child with the IgA deficiency, all children had normal for age serum concentrations of IgA, IgG, and IgM. Twenty-eight (43.0%) patients commenced daily treatment with ICS with or without LABA. Patients' clinical characteristics and their correlation with the prescription of ICS are shown in Table 1. Spirometry results and bacteria isolated from sputum cultures at the first and second visit are shown in Table 2. Dyspnea, presence of mosaic pattern, positive SPT, and positive BDR test were significantly correlated with the prescription of ICS (Table 1).

The multivariate logistic regression model included as explanatory variables the presence dyspnea, positive SPT, and of mosaic pattern, and corroborated the correlations found in univariate analysis between these variables and the decision to prescribe ICS (OR:5.35; CI:1.11, 25.80; $p = 0.036$, and OR:10.89; CI:2.21, 53.23; $p = 0.003$, and OR:12.55; CI:1.21, 121.61; $p = 0.034$, respectively). BDR test was not included in the model due to its small sample size and the lack of variation that did not allow a reliable estimation of model parameters. The three regression models showed that ICS use was not correlated with the differences in FEV1, FEV1/FVC, and the number of positive cultures, between the follow-up and the initial visit ($p = 0.29$, $p = 0.69$, and $p = 0.20$, respectively).

Table 1. Correlations of the main clinical, radiological, and laboratory characteristics of the 65 bronchiectasis patients with inhaled corticosteroids.

			Correlation with ICS Use	
	Without ICS Use ($n = 28$)	With ICS Use ($n = 37$)	Spearman ρ (CI)	p
Male, n (%)	16 (53.3)	14 (46.6)	0.08 (−0.22, 0.33)	0.90
Age at referral, years, n (%)	7.5 (2.7)	7.7 (2.8)	0.04 (−0.19, 0.29)	0.86
SPT, n (%)	28 (100)	37 (100)		
- Positive SPT, n (%)	1 (2.7)	15 (53.6)	0.55 (0.36, 0.70)	<0.001
Serum IgE, IU/mL, mean (sd)	49.8 (47.7)	72.1 (69.4)	0.25 (−0.03, 0.45)	0.16
Blood eosinophil count, mean (sd)	260 (225)	361 (322)	0.26 (0.01, 0.40)	0.20
T2-high status, n (%)	3 (8.1)	3 (10.7)	0.04 (−0.09–0.39)	0.72
Spirometry, n (%)	22 (48.9)	23 (51.1)		
- ppFEV1, mean (sd)	94.2 (13.5)	88.5 (12.1)	−0.41 (−0.63, −0.14)	0.13
- ppFVC, mean (sd)	92.9 (20.2)	88.1 (23.8)	−0.25 (−0.09, 0.78)	0.49
- FEV1/FVC, mean (sd)	87.1 (7.9)	83.9 (8.9)	−0.37 (−0.62, −0.13)	0.25
Bronchodilator response test, n (%)	10 (34.5)	19 (65.5)		
- Positive bronchodilator response test, n (%)	0 (0)	11 (57.9)	0.57 (0.21, 0.92)	0.001
Reported symptoms				
- Episodes of dyspnea, n (%)	4 (10.8)	18 (64.3)	0.55 (0.36, 0.70)	<0.001
- Wheezing, n (%)	8 (21.6)	15 (53.6)	0.33 (0.09, 0.53)	0.31
Modified Bhalla score, mean (sd)	4.1 (2.4)	3.6 (2.3)	0.21 (0.08, 0.42)	0.25
Mosaic pattern on HRCT, n (%)	12 (32.4)	24 (85.7)	0.53 (0.33, 0.68)	<0.001
Exacerbations during the first six months of treatment, median (IQR)	2 (1,2)	2 (1,3)	0.13 (0.02, 0.28)	0.27

ICS: Inhaled corticosteroids; HRCT: High-resolution computed tomography; SPT: Skin prick tests; pp: percent predicted.

Table 2. Spirometry results and bacteria isolated from sputum cultures at the first and second visit of patients.

	Initial Visit ($n = 65$)	Follow-Up Visit ($n = 65$)	p
Spirometry, n (%)	45 (69.2)	45 (69.2)	1
- ppFEV1, mean (sd)	91.8 (20.4)	93.1 (19.1)	0.65
- ppFVC, mean (sd)	90.1 (23.3)	93.3 (24.6)	0.44
- FEV1/FVC, mean (sd)	84.4 (10.4)	85.6 (11.5)	0.50
Positive sputum cultures, n (%)	38 (58.4)	3 (13.8)	<0.001
- Gram-negative bacteria, n	12	2	
- Staphylococcus aureus, n	7	1	
- Pseudomonas aeruginosa, n	7	0	
- Haemophilus influenzae, n	5	0	
- Streptococcus pneumoniae, n	4	0	
- Others, n	3	0	

4. Discussion

Many of the bronchiectatic patients in our study had clinical, and/or spirometry, and/or radiological findings indicative of airway obstruction which could be attributed either to coexisting asthma or to bronchiectasis per se. The lack of a simple test for the identification of asthma in children and the absence of strict criteria for ICS use in bronchiectasis, allow physicians to decide on the prescription of these drugs in a seemingly arbitrary way. Very often physicians base their diagnosis of asthma on a therapeutic trial of ICS and a careful assessment of the children's response. Unfortunately, this approach is not always helpful in patients with bronchiectasis due to the confounding effect of co-administered treatments. Some authors have suggested that ICS should be reserved for children with evidence of type 2–mediated allergic airway inflammation, whose existence can be roughly determined or ruled out by the measurements of eosinophils and IgE with or without concurrent measurement of fractional exhaled nitric oxide (FeNO) [8,12]. However, asthma in children is a heterogeneous disorder and atopic inflammation is neither necessary nor sufficient for its development. So, the aforementioned markers cannot be considered as definitive diagnostic tools for asthma [13]. In the present study, the main findings that influenced the decision of ICS prescription were the reported episodes of dyspnea, the presence of mosaic pattern on HRCT, the positive SPTs to aeroallergens, and the positive BDR test.

Dyspnea and wheezing were the only clinical signs/symptoms that were included in our analysis as they represent the two most common characteristics reported by parents, or experienced by children, with asthma [14]; only dyspnea was shown to affect the decision for ICS prescription. A probable explanation is that dyspnea is a rather unusual symptom in bronchiectasis, with a reported incidence ranging from 8.8–25.0% [3,15], while it is very common in asthma. On the other hand, wheeze implies flow limitation and it is not an exclusive characteristic of asthma. In bronchiectasis, it can be produced from mucus hypersecretion leading to bronchostenosis and the collapse of bronchial walls during expiration. Furthermore, when patients/parents report wheeze it is far from clear what they actually describe since many use this term for any noisy breathing [5,16].

Atopy, which is a considerable risk factor for asthma development [17,18], was investigated through SPT's to aeroallergens, as well as total serum IgE and absolute blood eosinophil count measurements. SPTs, which are strongly associated with respiratory allergy and asthma [19], were associated with ICS prescription. On the contrary, no significant association was found between ICS prescription and the serum IgE or eosinophil count, or their combination in a T_H2-high status variable. This may have resulted from serum IgE and eosinophil count being less consistent markers of asthma and allergy due to the absence of specific cut off values and the considerable overlap between normal and allergic patients [18,20].

Spirometry results were not a significant determinant of ICS prescription in our population. Indeed, spirometric values are usually normal in asthmatic children who are not in exacerbation and so they are not a reliable marker of asthma [21]. On the contrary, a positive BDR test has 50% positive predictive value in identifying response to ICS in asthmatic children with normal spirometry [22], and in accordance with this, our study showed the test to be a significant predictor of ICS prescription.

The mosaic pattern in expiration HRCT scans reflects air trapping and it is a well-known radiological feature of bronchiectasis [23]. However, air trapping was correlated with ICS prescription as it also represents a characteristic of asthma, with studies in adults and children having shown that it has a strong relationship with disease severity and peripheral airway obstruction [24,25].

The present study has certain limitations. The data depict the prescription preferences of physicians from a single centre and so the results are neither free from bias nor can be generalized. Cough, one of the main features of asthma, was not assessed because it is also the cardinal symptom of bronchiectasis and as such it could not offer any discriminative information for asthma diagnosis. HRCT scans were evaluated by a single radiologist and were not blinded. All children received antibiotics and started chest physiotherapy at diagnosis. Because of this, we were unable to determine the net result, if any, of ICS in children with asthma-like features. We tried to examine whether the administration of ICS could result in any measurable clinical changes that would allow us to identify a group of children who could truly benefit from ICS. However, since the study was not designed to investigate this question, included only a few outcome variables, and the sample size was relatively small, the results were inconclusive.

In conclusion, it was shown that the prescription of ICS in children with bronchiectasis is more likely when there are certain asthma-like features. The results should be conceptualized as a justification of the clinicians' decisions in cases where the coexistence of bronchiectasis and asthma seems probable and not as evidence for the need for ICS in certain cases. Indirectly, the study stresses the importance of research data able to illuminate the issue of asthma and bronchiectasis coexistence and define the clinical characteristics of children with bronchiectasis who could benefit from the use of ICS.

Author Contributions: K.D. and K.N.P. conceived and designed the study; K.D. analyzed the data and wrote the first draft of the manuscript; O.S., D.M. and A.G. collected the data; S.P., and E.A. reviewed and summarized the radiological data. All authors have read and agreed to the published version of the manuscript.

Funding: This research received no external funding.

Conflicts of Interest: The authors declare no conflict of interest.

References

1. Chang, A.B.; Bell, S.C.; Byrnes, C.A.; Grimwood, K.; Holmes, P.W.; King, P.T.; Kolbe, J.; Landau, L.I.; Maguire, G.P.; McDonald, M.I.; et al. Chronic suppurative lung disease and bronchiectasis in children and adults in Australia and New Zealand. A position statement from the Thoracic Society of Australia and New Zealand and the Australian Lung Foundation. *Med. J. Aust.* **2010**, *193*, 356–365. [CrossRef] [PubMed]
2. Santamaria, F.; Montella, S.; Pifferi, M.; Ragazzo, V.; De Stefano, S.; De Paulis, N.; Maglione, M.; Boner, A. A Descriptive Study of Non-Cystic Fibrosis Bronchiectasis in a Pediatric Population from Central and Southern Italy. *Respiration* **2009**, *77*, 160–165. [CrossRef] [PubMed]
3. Doğru, D.; Nik-Ain, A.; Kiper, N.; Göçmen, A.; Ozcelik, U.; Yalçın, E.; Aslan, A.T. Bronchiectasis: The Consequence of Late Diagnosis in Chronic Respiratory Symptoms. *J. Trop. Pediatr.* **2005**, *51*, 362–365. [CrossRef] [PubMed]
4. Douros, K.; Boutopoulou, B.; Papadopoulos, M.; Fouzas, S. Perception of dyspnea in children with asthma. *Front. Biosci. (Elite Ed.)* **2015**, *7*, 469–477. [CrossRef]
5. Priftis, K.N.; Douros, K.; Anthracopoulos, M.B. Snoring, hoarseness, stridor and wheezing. In *Paediatric Respiratory Medicine*; European Respiratory Society (ERS): Lausanne, Switzerland, 2013; pp. 57–64.
6. Crimi, C.; Ferri, S.; Crimi, N. Bronchiectasis and asthma. *Curr. Opin. Allergy Clin. Immunol.* **2019**, *19*, 46–52. [CrossRef]
7. Chang, A.B.; Bell, S.C.; Torzillo, P.J.; King, P.T.; Maguire, G.P.; Byrnes, C.A.; Holland, A.E.; O'Mara, P.; Grimwood, K. Chronic suppurative lung disease and bronchiectasis in children and adults in Australia and New Zealand Thoracic Society of Australia and New Zealand guidelines. *Med. J. Aust.* **2015**, *202*, 21–23. [CrossRef]

8. Chang, A.B.; Bush, A.; Grimwood, K. Bronchiectasis in children: Diagnosis and treatment. *Lancet* **2018**, *392*, 866–879. [CrossRef]
9. Kapur, N.; Masel, J.P.; Watson, D.; Masters, I.B.; Chang, A.B. Bronchoarterial Ratio on High-Resolution CT Scan of the Chest in Children Without Pulmonary Pathology. *Chest* **2011**, *139*, 1445–1450. [CrossRef]
10. Castile, R.; Long, F.; Flucke, R.; Goldstein, A.; Filbrun, D.; Brody, A.; McCoy, K. High resolution computed tomography of the chest in infants with cystic fibrosis. *Pediatr. Pulmonol.* **1999**, *19*, 401.
11. Tran, T.N.; Zeiger, R.S.; Peters, S.P.; Colice, G.; Newbold, P.; Goldman, M.; Chipps, B.E. Overlap of atopic, eosinophilic, and TH2-high asthma phenotypes in a general population with current asthma. *Ann. Allergy Asthma Immunol.* **2016**, *116*, 37–42. [CrossRef]
12. Licari, A.; Manti, S.; Castagnoli, R.; Leonardi, S.; Marseglia, G.L. Measuring inflammation in paediatric severe asthma: Biomarkers in clinical practice. *Breathe* **2020**, *16*, 190301. [CrossRef] [PubMed]
13. Anthracopoulos, M.B.; Dm, M.L.E. Asthma: A Loss of Post-natal Homeostatic Control of Airways Smooth Muscle with Regression Toward a Pre-natal State. *Front. Pediatr.* **2020**, *8*, 95. [CrossRef] [PubMed]
14. Yoos, H.L.; Kitzman, H.; McMullen, A.; Sidora-Arcoleo, K.; Anson, E. The language of breathlessness: Do families and health care providers speak the same language when describing asthma symptoms? *J. Pediatr. Health Care* **2005**, *19*, 197–205. [CrossRef] [PubMed]
15. Kim, H.-Y.; Kwon, J.; Seo, J.; Song, Y.-H.; Kim, B.-J.; Yu, J.; Hong, S. Bronchiectasis in Children: 10-Year Experience at a Single Institution. *Allergy Asthma Immunol. Res.* **2011**, *3*, 39–45. [CrossRef] [PubMed]
16. Douros, K.; Dm, M.L.E. Time to Say Goodbye to Bronchiolitis, Viral Wheeze, Reactive Airways Disease, Wheeze Bronchitis and All That. *Front. Pediatr.* **2020**, *8*, 218. [CrossRef]
17. Weinmayr, G.; Weiland, S.K.; Björkstén, B.; Brunekreef, B.; Büchele, G.; Cookson, W.O.C.; Garcia-Marcos, L.; Gotua, M.; Gratziou, C.; Van Hage, M.; et al. Atopic Sensitization and the International Variation of Asthma Symptom Prevalence in Children. *Am. J. Respir. Crit. Care Med.* **2007**, *176*, 565–574. [CrossRef] [PubMed]
18. Weinmayr, G.; Genuneit, J.; Nagel, G.; Björkstén, B.; Van Hage, M.; Priftanji, A.; Cooper, P.; Rijkjärv, M.-A.; Von Mutius, E.; Tsanakas, J.; et al. International variations in associations of allergic markers and diseases in children: ISAAC Phase Two. *Allergy* **2009**, *65*, 766–775. [CrossRef]
19. Moustaki, M.; Loukou, I.; Tsabouri, S.; Douros, K. The Role of Sensitization to Allergen in Asthma Prediction and Prevention. *Front. Pediatr.* **2017**, *5*, 166. [CrossRef]
20. Klink, M.; Cline, M.G.; Halonen, M.; Burrows, B. Problems in defining normal limits for serum IgE. *J. Allergy Clin. Immunol.* **1990**, *85*, 440–444. [CrossRef]
21. Bacharier, L.B.; Strunk, R.C.; Mauger, D.; White, D.; Lemanske, R.F.; Sorkness, C.A. Classifying Asthma Severity in Children. *Am. J. Respir. Crit. Care Med.* **2004**, *170*, 426–432. [CrossRef]
22. Galant, S.P.; Morphew, T.; Guijon, O.; Pham, L. The bronchodilator response as a predictor of inhaled corticosteroid responsiveness in asthmatic children with normal baseline spirometry. *Pediatr. Pulmonol.* **2014**, *49*, 1162–1169. [CrossRef] [PubMed]
23. Edwards, E.A.; Metcalfe, R.; Milne, D.G.; Thompson, J.; Byrnes, C.A. Retrospective review of children presenting with non cystic fibrosis bronchiectasis: HRCT features and clinical relationships. *Pediatr. Pulmonol.* **2003**, *36*, 87–93. [CrossRef] [PubMed]
24. Jain, N.; Covar, R.A.; Gleason, M.C.; Newell, J.D.; Gelfand, E.W.; Spahn, J.D. Quantitative computed tomography detects peripheral airway disease in asthmatic children. *Pediatr. Pulmonol.* **2005**, *40*, 211–218. [CrossRef] [PubMed]
25. De Blic, J.; Scheinmann, P. The use of imaging techniques for assessing severe childhood asthma. *J. Allergy Clin. Immunol.* **2007**, *119*, 808–810. [CrossRef]

Publisher's Note: MDPI stays neutral with regard to jurisdictional claims in published maps and institutional affiliations.

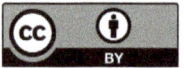

© 2020 by the authors. Licensee MDPI, Basel, Switzerland. This article is an open access article distributed under the terms and conditions of the Creative Commons Attribution (CC BY) license (http://creativecommons.org/licenses/by/4.0/).

MDPI
St. Alban-Anlage 66
4052 Basel
Switzerland
Tel. +41 61 683 77 34
Fax +41 61 302 89 18
www.mdpi.com

Journal of Clinical Medicine Editorial Office
E-mail: jcm@mdpi.com
www.mdpi.com/journal/jcm

www.ingramcontent.com/pod-product-compliance
Lightning Source LLC
LaVergne TN
LVHW070045120526
838202LV00101B/540